HOW TO STAY FIT AND HEALTHY

ARVIND UPADHYAY

ISBN 979-888546956-2

Congratulations on taking a forward step to get in shape and feel great. Many people are guilty of wishing they could get a sculpted body from eating junk food and watching TV all day. But that is just not going to happen. Even though getting in shape sounds like a long, time-wasting process, the effort put towards being in shape has many positive effects. If you want to start your journey to having a better body to feel great, here are some tips:

1. Exercise Daily

Exercise daily for at least an hour. You do not have to kill yourself from running, jogging, etc., but you should have some sort of moderate physical activity in your everyday life. If you're looking to shed a few pounds fast, do a higher-level intensity workout. For example, go on a walk at a brisk pace for an hour. Or, you can jog and set certain intervals to sprint during that hour. Make sure you're not in severe pain during your workout. Just a warning, your muscles will ache after a high intensity workout. It may be irritating, but that means your body is changing for the better. Be sure to stay hydrated, stretch, and eat foods with a decent amount of protein after each workout. The protein will help keep your muscles, not fat, rebuilding.

2. Eat the Right Foods and Portion Each Meal

No matter how bad your stomach is telling you to go for candy over healthy food, try to stay away from sweets. Sugar from candy will not help you get in shape. Even if it's just a single candy bar, one will eventually lead to another. Fruits and vegetables are the best thing to eat when getting into shape. Apples, for example, do a good job at making the stomach feel full for up to 3 to 4 hours. Green vegetables such as green beans and broccoli keep the digestive system clean and running.

Also, stick to lean meats like turkey and chicken. Seafood, such as, shrimp, and tilapia are also great alternatives. These foods are full of protein and healthy nutrients to help keep muscles fit and ready for workouts. In addition, be sure to portion what you eat. Having a good metabolism comes from portioning meals. Try to plan out eating six times a day and setting smaller portions, rather than having three large meals throughout the day. This will also help you find yourself breathing smoother when working out rather than huffing and puffing for air. This is because you will have less food in your digestive system, which means more energy is used toward your exercise.

3. Keep Track of Calories and Food Intake Per Day

Keeping track of how many calories you eat in a day will be helpful in planning out your physical exercising. Ever wonder why body builders' body masses are so big? That's because they plan out their meals and take in more (healthy) calories than the average person. On the other hand, losing weight and striving for a skinnier physique will involve more physical exercise than calories you ingest.

4. Be Sure to Get Sleep

Even though most of us have eight-hour jobs during the day or night, it is crucial to get enough sleep to recharge the body's batteries. Six to eight hours of sleep will keep the body going throughout the day, but if you happen to feel tired at any point after coming home from work, by all means take a small nap before exercising. You should only nap for about a half hour. This will prevent you from staying up later in the night.

5. Stay Motivated

An important key to being in shape is to set goals and keep a positive mindset. If you stay positive, you will be able to push yourself to get that fit body you've always wanted.

Erie Cross Training Examiner Kyle Melerski, a music technology student at Capital University, is on the rise by using his creative writing skills to inform and entertain people.

Examiner.com is the inside source for everything local. Powered by Examiners, the largest pool of knowledgeable and passionate contributors in the world, we provide unique and original content to enhance life in your local city wherever that may be.

Before explaining what a physical fitness program should look like, there are some basic terms that must be discussed. These principals apply to all programs in general and must be addressed in the development of any fitness program. INTENSITY — The amount of effort put into each workout, usually measured by heartbeats per minute. For the maximum benefit in each workout, plan on exercising at a minimum of 70 percent of the heart rate reserve. There are several scientific ways to your heart rate reserve. The simplest way is to begin with you maximum heart rate (220-Age). Next, measure your resting heart rate. The heart rate reserve is found by Max heart rate - resting heart rate. To train at 70% of the heart rate reserve you would multiply 70% by the heart rate reserve and then add your resting heart rate. For a 20 year old with a resting heart rate of 60 to dDetermineing your training heart rate in beats per minute would be 70% x Heart Rate Reserve =.70 x (200-60) + 60 (Resting Heart Rate) = a training heart rate of 158 beats per min. DURATION – The length each exercise period should last. There has been a great deal of research on this topic. Most experts believe that when working on your cardiovascular endurance a minimum of 20 to 30 minutes is needed to obtain maximum benefit. This holds true for the majority of the population. The only notable exception occurs for long distance or endurance athletes (e.g. marathon runners or triathletes). FREQUENCY – The number of workouts one should have per week. Once again experts agree that the average person requires a minimum of three workouts per week to improve their current level of fitness. Working out less frequently will only maintain a level of fitness; it will not improve the level of fitness. When exercising only three times a week, each period should be medium to high intensity. Exercising with consistent frequency can also be referred to as REGULARITY. Exercise must be done regularly to produce a training effect. Sporadic exercise may cause more harm in the form of injury than benefit from exercise. The same is true for extremely intense workouts. They may create injuries. RECOVERY – Do not work the same muscle groups hard day after day. Muscles need recovery time. People frequently misunderstand this point. Providing inadequate recovery can explain the reason why most people see little or no gain from excessive exercise. You can work the same muscle groups each day, however, you should work hard one day and easy the next. This is a critical point because this fitness program is based on a six days a week exercise program. GENERAL ADAPTATION PRINCIPAL (GAP) – Muscles as well as your cardiovascular system in the body will adapt to the increasing stress placed upon it through exercise. To see gains in a fitness program one must stress the existing muscular and cardiovascular systems. This can also be called the OVERLOAD principal. For a muscle to increase in strength, the workload during exercise must be larger than what it normally experiences. 5 SPECIFICITY – There are several different exercises and events that can develop your muscular strength as well as cardiovascular fitness. To increase the number of push-ups you can do, simply increase upper body strength through a number of strength exercises and weights. However, the best way to improve push-ups requires doing push-ups. Similarly one can improve cardiovascular fitness by biking swimming, or walking. However, if the goal remains an improved ability to run, the best exercise will be running. MAJOR COMPONENTS OF PHYSICAL FITNESS – There are several components of any fitness program. The three major components of most programs are flexibility, strength, muscular endurance, and cardiovascular endurance. These components are the essential elements of the Army Physical Fitness Program. How to Use These Workout Programs These programs are designed as four week plans. Each program has a workout A & B. Alternate workouts daily for 6 days, then rest. For example, perform workout A on Monday, Wednesday, and Friday; perform workout B on Tuesday, Thursday, and Saturday. Different muscles are trained in workouts A & B, which means you are training each muscle group 3 days per week. Rest Sunday. Work cardiovascular exercises into your workouts at least 3 times per week. You may attempt to eventually work up to doing cardio 6 days a week using the hard/easy technique mentioned under the recovery principle. Fitness Assessment Before starting any new fitness program it is important to assess ones abilities. This includes knowing strengths as well as weaknesses. Ideally, a fitness program would improve weak areas and maintain or improve strength areas. However, before explaining the diagnostic test there are other important factors and preferences that should be identified. These factors and preferences may include the time of day to workout, how much time is available each day to workout, individual or team sports, and finally the goal of the fitness program. The questionnaire attached is intended to give a fitness trainer the basics they need to personalize a fitness program that will works.

Contents

Foreword   *ix*

  1. The Complete Fitness   1

  2. Easy Way To Get Fit   27

  3. Intelligent Person's Guide To Fitness   32

  4. Strength Training   50

  5. How To Stay Fit Forever: 25 Tips To Keep Moving When Life   69
     Gets In The Way

  6. No Gym Required: How To Get Fit At Home Get In Shape   76
     Without Leaving The House

  7. Endurance Training   82

  8. Nutrition   99

  9. Weight Management   127

 10. Special Exercises For Special People   137

Ways To Stay Fit And Healthy   163

Foreword

Your physical fitness is your ability to perform physical work, training, and other activities throughout your daily work schedule. Physical fitness is multidimensional, and—based on your goals—some components will be more valuable than others. Five key components define your physical fitness: • Cardiorespiratory (CR) endurance—how efficiently your body delivers oxygen and nutrients for muscular activity and transports waste from the cells • Muscular strength—the greatest amount of force your muscle or muscle group can exert in a single effort • Muscular endurance—the ability of your muscle or muscle group to perform repeated movements for extended periods • Flexibility—the ability to move your joints (elbow or knee, for example) or any group of joints through their entire normal range of motion • Body composition—the amount of body fat you have in comparison with your total body mass. Improving the first three of these components will improve your body composition by decreasing your body fat. Excessive body fat detracts from the other fitness measures, reduces your physical and mental performance, detracts from your appearance, and increases overall health risks. One measurement of body fat is as a percentage of your total weight. The Army's maximum allowable percentages of body fat, by age and gender, are listed in Figure 2.1. Besides your physical fitness, you should also work to improve your motor fitness. Motor fitness—speed, agility, muscle power, eye-hand coordination, and eye-foot coordination— directly affect a Soldier's performance on the battlefield. Appropriate training will improve these elements up to each Soldier's individual potential. The goal of the Army's fitness program is to improve physical and motor fitness through sound, progressive, mission-specific physical training at both the individual and unit levels.

Practicing the basic exercise principles is crucial for you to develop an effective fitnesstraining program. The principles of exercise apply to everyone at all levels of physical training, from the Olympic champion to the weekend golfer. They apply especially to fitness training for military personnel because having standard fitness principles across the organization saves time, energy, resources—and prevents injury. You can easily remember the basic principles of exercise if you recall the P-R-O-V-RB-S acronym: 78 ■ SECTION 2 Figure 2.1 Body Fat Standards P-R-O-V-R-B-S the basic exercise principles—Progression, Regularity, Overload,

Variety, Recovery, Balance, and Specificity 8420010_PD2_p076-085 8/14/ 08 10:42 AM Page 78 P Progression—The intensity and duration of exercise must gradually increase to improve your fitness level. A good guideline for improvement is a 10 percent gain at specified intervals. R Regularity—To achieve effective training you should schedule workouts in each of the first four fitness components at least three times a week. Regularity is also key in resting, sleeping, and following a good diet. O Overload—The workload of each exercise session must exceed the normal demands placed on your body to bring about a training effect. You've often heard this expressed as "No pain, no gain." A fitness trainer, such as your ROTC instructor, can help you learn to tell the difference between pain that results from an optimum level of overload and pain that indicates potential injury. V Variety—Changing activities reduces the boredom and increases your motivation to progress. R Recovery—You should follow a hard day of training for a given component of fitness by an easier training or rest day for that component. This helps your body recover. Another way to promote recovery is to alternate the muscle groups you exercise every other day, especially when training for strength and muscle endurance. B Balance—To be effective, a fitness program should address all the fitness components, since overemphasizing any one of them may detract from the others. S Specificity—You must gear training toward specific goals. For example, Soldiers become better runners if their training emphasizes running drills and techniques. Although swimming is great exercise, it will not improve a two-mile-run time as much as a coordinated running program does.

CHAPTER ONE

THE COMPLETE FITNESS

(1) Equipment. Flat weight bench. At least 1, preferably 2 spotters. Lifting gloves are authorized. Bench press shirts are not authorized. (2) Performance. Lie in a supine position on a flat bench with your legs positioned at the sides of the bench and your feet flat on the floor. Using a handgrip that is about 6 inches wider than your shoulder width, bring the barbell to arms length above the chest but in line with the shoulders (see fig 1). If two spotters are available they will position themselves on each side of the bar. The spotters may assist in the liftoff. If only one spotter is available, he/she will be at the lifter's head to assist. Once the bar is at the start position the spotter will release the bar. Lower the barbell to the chest and make a definite pause. As soon as momentum has ceased the grader will yell press. Press the barbell to the start position to complete the repetition. The spotter will not touch the barbell during the repetition 8 unless absolutely necessary. If the spotter has to assist the lifter during the repetition the event is terminated. Upper Body Strength = 1 rep max in pounds divided by body weight in pounds Males Females 5 greater than 1.26 5 greater than .78 4 1.17 - 1.25 4 .72 - .77 3 .97 - 1.16 3 .59 - .71 2 .88 - .96 2 .53 - .58 1 less than .87 1 less than .52 2. Second Event: Push-up. Cadets will perform as many push-ups as they can to determine the muscular endurance of the chest shoulder, and triceps muscles. (1) Equipment. Flat area. (2) Performance. On the command 'get set,' assume the front-leaning rest position by placing your hands where they are comfortable for you. Your feet may be together or up to 12 inches apart. When viewed from the side, your body should form a generally straight line from your shoulders to your ankles. On the command 'go,' begin the push-up by bending your elbows and lowering your entire body as a single unit until your upper arms are at least parallel to the ground. Then, return to the starting position by raising your entire body until your arms are fully extended. Your body must

remain rigid in a generally straight line and move as a unit while performing each repetition. At the end of each repetition, the scorer will state the number of repetitions you have completed correctly. If you fail to keep your body generally straight, to lower your whole body until your upper arms are at least parallel to the ground, or to extend your arms completely, that repetition will not count, and the scorer will repeat the number of the last correctly performed repetition. An altered, front-leaning rest position is the only authorized rest position. That is, you may sag in the middle or flex your back. When flexing your back, you may bend your knees, but not to such an extent that you are supporting most of your body weight with your legs. If this occurs, your performance will be terminated. You must return to, and pause in, the correct starting position before continuing. If you rest on the ground or raise either hand or foot from the ground, your performance will be terminated. You may reposition your hands and/or feet during the event as long as they remain in contact with the ground at all times. Correct performance is important. You will do as many push-ups as you can; there is no time limit. 3. Third Event: Curl-up. Cadets will perform the curl-up exercise to assess abdominal strength and endurance. (1) Equipment. Mat, Ruler, metronome, stop watch (2) Performance. Start with your back on the floor with your knees bent at a 90 degree angle (feet 12 to 18 inches away from the buttocks). Place your arms by your sides with palms down on the floor, elbows locked, and fingers straight. The grader will place a ruler or draw a line 12 cm away from the longest finger tip and set metronome to a cadence of 50 beats per 9 minute. Curl your head and upper back upward, keeping arms stiff, reaching forward along the floor to touch the line. Your fingers, feet and buttocks must stay on the floor during the entire curl-up. Slide the palms of the hands (extended arms) along the mat until the fingertips of both hands just touch the 12 cm line. Keep the arms straight. Lower your body until the back is flat against the ground. Perform the movement following the cadence of the metronome (25 curl-ups per minute). Take the same amount of time to perform the raising and lowering phases. The test score is the number of complete touches on the line until the rhythm cannot be followed. If you do not have a Metronome, conduct standard bent knee sit-ups with your hands crossed over your chest. Do as many as you can in a 2 minute period. Male AGE 15-19 20-29 30-39 Excellent >74 >74 >74 Above Average 35 - 74 31 - 74 36 - 74 Average 24 - 34 24 - 30 26 - 35 Below Average 8 - 23 4 - 23 0 - 23 Female AGE 15-19 20-29 30-39 Excellent >74 >69 >54 Above Average 30 -

74 30 - 69 28 - 54 Average 24 - 29 21 - 29 15 - 27 Below Average 10 - 23 5 - 20 0 - 14 Fourth Event: Step Test. Cadets will perform the 3-minute step test to determine cardiovascular endurance. (1) Equipment. Metronome, 12 inch step, stopwatch. (2) Performance. Cadets will step up (1-2) and down (3-4) in cadence with the metronome which is set at 96 beats per minute (4 clicks = one step cycle) for a stepping rate of 24 steps per minute. Cadets will step up and down on the 12-inch bench for 3 minutes. Immediately after the 3-minute stepping exercise, the cadet is to sit down and within 5 seconds, the tester is to take the subject's heart rate for one minute. The total one-minute post-exercise heart rate is the subject's score for the test. Compare to YMCA Norms below. In the event you do not have a Metronome, the tester will count one step-two step-three step-four step in an attempt to come close to 96 beats per minute. Needless to say, this will result in a less accurate evaluation. Example: A 18- year old female performs the step test with a final heart rate of 95. Looking at the table she falls under the above average profile. 10 Physical Fitness Evaluation on Profile for 3-Minute Step Test (Heart Rate values in beats per minute) MALE AGE 18-25 26-35 36-45 Classification Excellent 70-78 73-79 72-81 Good 79-88 80-88 82-94 Above Average 89-97 89-97 95-102 Average 98-104 98-106 103-111 Below Average 105-114 109-116 112-118 Poor 115-128 117-126 119-128 Very Poor 129-164 127-164 129-168 FEMALE AGE 18-25 26-35 36-45 Classification Excellent 70-78 73-79 72-81 Good 79-88 80-88 82-94 Above Average 89-97 89-97 95-102 Average 98-104 98-106 103-111 Below Average 105-114 109-116 112-118 Poor 115-128 117-126 119-128 Very Poor 129-164 127-164 129-168 11 5. Fifth Event: Sit & Reach. Cadets will perform the sit and reach to determine hamstring and lower back flexibility. (1) Equipment. Ruler. (2) Performance. Sit on the floor with legs out straight ahead and shoes off. The tester holds both knees flat against the floor. Lean forward slowly as far as possible and hold the greatest stretch for two seconds. Make sure there is no jerky movements, and that the fingertips remain level and the legs flat. The score is recorded as the distance before (negative) or beyond (positive) from the toes. Repeat twice and record the best score. The table below (figure 3) gives you a guide for expected scores in cm for adults. Men (cm from toes) Women (cm from toes) Super > +27 > +30 Excellent +17 to +27 +21 to +30 Good +6 to +16 +11 to +20 Average 0 to +5 +1 to +10 Fair -8 to −1 -7 to 0 Poor -19 to -9 -14 to -8 Very poor < -20 < -15 12 6. Sixth Event: Illinois Agility Run Test. Cadets will perform the Illinois Agility Run Test to test agility.

(1) Equipment. flat surface (minimum 20m x10m area), 8 cones, a stop watch. (2) Course. The length of the course is 10 meters and the width (distance between the start and finish points) is 5 meters. On the track you could use 5 lanes. 4 cones can be used to mark the start, finish and the two turning points. Each cone in the center is spaced 3.3 meters apart. Gender Excellent Above Average Average Below Average Poor Male 18.3 secs Female 23.0 secs 13 Administration. Professors of Military Science & Leadership (PMS) should administer the diagnostic test in the assessment phase of the fitness program development. Use the Diagnostic Test Score Card provided. The next diagnostic test should occur no later than week six. Subsequent diagnostic tests should be given every six weeks. After the initial diagnostic it is acceptable to substitute the APFT as a diagnostic tool. PMSs or their designated fitness expert should regularly monitor the fitness logs of cadets and provide guidance as needed. Diagnostic Test Score Card Last Name First Name MI Gender M or F Age Height ______inches Weight _______lbs Body Fat _______% Bench Press Lift 1______ 2______ 3______ 4______ 5______ 1-RM = lbs 1 Rep Maximum Divided by Bodyweight = Push-up Repetitions________ Curl-up Repetitions________ Step Test 1-minute post-exercise heart rate _______beats Sit & Reach Distance from toes (+ or -) ________cm Illinois Agility Run Test Time_____________ 14 Flexibility Flexibility is an important component of your fitness program. Many activity- related injuries have their root in lack of flexibility. Think of your muscles as rubber bands. When they are cold they are rigid and brittle. When warm they stretch and retract more easily. Conducting a good warm-up prior to exercising and a good cool-down upon completion will help prevent injury and reduce muscle soreness. No matter what your current fitness level, you should always begin your exercise sessions with a warm-up. A good warm-up sequence is as follows. Jog in place or a specified location for one to two minutes. This causes a gradual increase in the heart rate, blood pressure, circulation, and increases the temperature of the active muscles. Next, perform slow joint rotation exercises (for example, arm circles, knee/ankle rotations) to gradually increase the joint's range of motion. Work each major joint for 5 to 10 seconds. Finally, stretch the muscles to be used during the upcoming activity slowly. This will "loosen up" muscles and tendons so they can achieve greater ranges of motion with less risk of injury. Hold each stretch position for 10 to 15 seconds, and do not bounce or bob. Immediately following your exercise session stretch as part of your cool-down. After exercising, when your muscles are their

warmest is the best time to improve your flexibility. Do not limit flexibility exercises to warm-up and cool-down only. Take the time to dedicate sessions to flexibility. Stretching throughout the day is also a great idea. Stretching is one form of exercise that takes very little time relative to the benefits gained. Some of the more common flexibility exercises are listed under the flexibility exercises. Assume all stretching positions slowly until you feel tension or slight discomfort. Hold each position for at least 10 to 15 seconds during the warm-up and cool-down. Developmental stretching to improve flexibility requires holding each stretch for 30 seconds or longer. 15 PROGRAM DESCRIPTION These Fitness Work-out sheets are designed to be implemented on a workout plan A followed the next day by a workout plan B. Workout A will focus on lower body strength and endurance while workout plan B will focus on upper body strength and endurance. Both days incorporate some abdominal work. Remember it is important to maintain a period of recovery for the abdominal muscles. Trying to overachieve early in a workout program can lead to injury. The reason there is a range within the abdominal exercises is to promote recovery. If you are providing yourself adequate time to recover, over time you should see your abilities increasing. The cardiorespiratory workouts need to be included into the program. If the program selected is exclusively running (e.g. group run, fartlek, or interval) it should replace the A workout plan. However, if you choose a guerrilla or grass drill workout plan it could substitute for either the A or the B Workout plan. The minimum frequency of cardiorespiratory workouts is two to three per week. For borderline runners the number of workouts may be as high as three to five per week and may consist of a combination of intervals, grass, and guerrilla drills. The determining factor for the intensity and frequency of cardiorespiratory training will depend on the ability and fitness level of the cadet and the intensity of the workout. For some reason if you miss A workout then the next workout would be the A workout. In a week you should expect to do a total of six workouts per week. 16 The Road to Fitness WORKOUT A EXERCISE WEEK 1 WEEK 2 WEEK 3 WEEK 4 SQUAT Weight/Reps Weight/Reps Weight/Reps Weight/Reps Set 1 12-15 reps / / / / Set 2 12-15 reps / / / / Set 3 12-15 reps / / / / LEG CURLS Weight/Reps Weight/Reps Weight/Reps Weight/Reps Set 1 12-15 reps / / / / Set 2 12-15 reps / / / / Set 3 12-15 reps / / / / Deadlifts Weight/Reps Weight/Reps Weight/Reps Weight/Reps Set 1 12-15 reps / / / / Set 2 12-15 reps / / / / Set 3 12-15 reps / / / / LEG EXTENSION Weight/Reps Weight/Reps Weight/Reps Weight/Reps Set 1 12-15 reps / /

/ / Set 2 12-15 reps / / / / Set 3 12-15 reps / / / / CALF RAISES Weight/ Reps Weight/Reps Weight/Reps Weight/Reps Set 1 12-15 reps / / / / Set 2 12-15 reps / / / / Set 3 12-15 reps / / / / ABDOMINAL SIT-UP 1 minute SWISS-BALL CRUNCH 1 minute REVERSE CRUNCH 1 minute Beginner Routine: Do one set of 12-15 reps of each exercise. Use a weight that you can lift at least 12 times. When you complete 15 reps, increase the weight at your next workout. Move quickly from exercise to exercise, resting at most 30 seconds between exercises unless you are exceeding your training heart rate. If you are, increase the rest period between exercises. As you progress, you should be able to decrease the rest between exercises while maintaining your training heart rate. SPEED: Perform each rep deliberately slower than what seems like your natural speed. This keeps your muscles under tension longer and helps build them faster. 17 The Road to Fitness WORKOUT B EXERCISE WEEK 1 WEEK 2 WEEK 3 WEEK 4 BENCH PRESS Weight/Reps Weight/Reps Weight/Reps Weight/Reps Set 1 12-15 reps / / / / Set 2 12-15 reps / / / / Set 3 12-15 reps / / / / INCLINE BENCH PRESS Weight/Reps Weight/Reps Weight/Reps Weight/Reps Set 1 12-15 reps / / / / Set 2 12-15 reps / / / / Set 3 12-15 reps / / / / DUMBELL SHOULDER PRESS Weight/Reps Weight/Reps Weight/Reps Weight/Reps Set 1 12-15 reps / / / / Set 2 12-15 reps / / / / Set 3 12-15 reps / / / / LATERAL RAISES Weight/Reps Weight/Reps Weight/Reps Weight/Reps Set 1 12-15 reps / / / / Set 2 12-15 reps / / / / Set 3 12-15 reps / / / / DIPS Weight/Reps Weight/Reps Weight/Reps Weight/Reps Set 1 12-15 reps / / / / Set 2 12-15 reps / / / / Set 3 12-15 reps / / / / ABDOMINAL WEIGHTED SIT-UP 15-25 REVERSE CRUNCH 15-25 BODY TWIST 15-25 Beginner Goals: Exercise consistently with short focused workouts. Build endurance through high-repetition strength training and moderate intensity cardiovascular exercise. See rapid increases in strength and modest gains in muscle mass. Advanced Goals: You'll focus more energy on strength training. Help your body recover from nagging injuries with short, low volume routines. You should leave the gym feeling as if you could have done a lot more. Give your muscle building systems a boost responding from a higher-volume routine to a change in volume. 18 Increase Muscle Mass WORKOUT A EXERCISE WEEK 1 WEEK 2 WEEK 3 WEEK 4 Leg Press Weight/Reps Weight/Reps Weight/Reps Weight/Reps Set 1 12-15 / / / / Set 2 12-15 / / / / Set 3 12-15 / / / / Lunges Weight/Reps Weight/Reps Weight/Reps Weight/Reps Set 1 12-15 / / / / Set 2 12-15 / / / / Set 3 12-15 / / / / Leg Curls Weight/Reps Weight/Reps Weight/Reps Weight/

Reps Set 1 12-15 / / / / Set 2 12-15 / / / / Set 3 12-15 / / / / Leg Extensions Weight/Reps Weight/Reps Weight/Reps Weight/Reps Set 1 12-15 / / / / Set 2 12-15 / / / / Set 3 12-15 / / / / Seated Calves Weight/Reps Weight/Reps Weight/Reps Weight/Reps Set 1 12-15 / / / / Set 2 12-15 / / / / Set 3 12-15 / / / / ABDOMINAL Crunch Circuit 25-30 Oblique Crunches 30-40 each side Superman 20-25 19 Increase Muscle Mass WORKOUT B EXERCISE WEEK 1 WEEK 2 WEEK 3 WEEK 4 CHEST Triset 1 Weight/Reps Weight/Reps Weight/Reps Weight/Reps Incline Dumbbell Bench / / / / Flat Dumbbell Bench / / / / Decline Dumbbell Bench / / / / BACK Triset 2 Weight/Reps Weight/Reps Weight/Reps Weight/Reps Lat Pull Down / / / / Upright Row / / / / Straight Arm Lat Pulldown / / / / SHOULDER Triset 3 Weight/Reps Weight/Reps Weight/Reps Weight/Reps Dumbbell Shoulder Press / / / / Cleans / / / / Seated Bent Over Row / / / / ARM/BICEPS Triset 4 Weight/Reps Weight/Reps Weight/Reps Weight/Reps Standing Bicep Curl / / / / Preacher Curl / / / / Hammer-Grip Bicep Curl / / / / ARM/TRICEPS Triset 5 Weight/Reps Weight/Reps Weight/Reps Weight/Reps Tricep Pushdown / / / / French Curls / / / / Tricep Kickbacks / / / / ABDOMINAL Crunch Circuit 25-30 Oblique Crunches 30-40 each side Superman 20-25 Beginner Goals: Perform equal volumes of work for all upper-body parts to strengthen stabilizer muscles. Start to see significant increases in muscle size and definition. Combine cardiovascular training with resistance training to maximize benefit. Advanced Goals: Bolster upper-body muscle and strength with multiple upper-body workouts in the same week. Increase your body's ability to tolerate max cardiovascular effort in order to improve endurance and increase metabolism. 20 Get Stronger WORKOUT A EXERCISE WEEK 1 WEEK 2 WEEK 3 WEEK 4 Squats Weight/Reps Weight/Reps Weight/Reps Weight/Reps Warm-up Set 1&2 6 reps / / / / Set 3 5-8 reps / / / / Set 4 5-8 reps / / / / Set 5 5-8 reps / / / / Lunges Weight/Reps Weight/Reps Weight/Reps Weight/Reps Warm-up Set 1&2 6 reps / / / / Set 3 5-8 reps / / / / Set 4 5-8 reps / / / / Set 5 5-8 reps / / / / Leg Curls Weight/Reps Weight/Reps Weight/Reps Weight/Reps Warm-up Set 1&2 6 reps / / / / Set 3 5-8 reps / / / / Set 4 5-8 reps / / / / Set 5 5-8 reps / / / / Leg Extensions Weight/Reps Weight/Reps Weight/Reps Weight/Reps Warm-up Set 1&2 6 reps / / / / Set 3 5-8 reps / / / / Set 4 5-8 reps / / / / Set 5 5-8 reps / / / / Seated Calves Weight/Reps Weight/Reps Weight/Reps Weight/Reps Warm-up Set 1&2 6 reps / / / / Set 3 5-8 reps / / / / Set 4 5-8 reps / / / / Set 5 5-8 reps / / / / ABDOMINAL Sit-ups 90 sec max Weighted sit-ups 45 sec max Incline sit-ups 30 sec max 21 Get Stronger in 4 WEEKS WORKOUT B EXERCISE WEEK 1 WEEK 2 WEEK 3 WEEK 4 ROPE CLIMB Set 1 30 FT Set 2 (Drop) 20 FT CURL AND PRESS Weight/Reps Weight/Reps Weight/Reps Weight/Reps Set 1 15 reps / / / / Set 2 (Drop) 10 reps / / / / LATERAL RAISE Weight/Reps Weight/Reps Weight/Reps Weight/Reps Set 1 15 reps / / / / Set 2 (Drop) 10 reps / / / / 90-Degree Lateral Raise Weight/Reps Weight/Reps Weight/Reps Weight/ Reps Set 1 15 reps / / / / Set 2 (Drop) 10 reps / / / / Dumbell Shoulder Press Weight/Reps Weight/Reps Weight/Reps Weight/Reps Set 1 15 reps / / / / Set 2 (Drop) 10 reps / / / / Lateral Raise Weight/Reps Weight/ Reps Weight/Reps Weight/Reps Set 1 15 reps / / / / Set 2 (Drop) 10 reps / / / / Dumbell Row Weight/Reps Weight/Reps Weight/Reps Weight/ Reps Set 1 15 reps / / / / Set 2 (Drop) 10 reps / / / / Triceps Kickback Weight/Reps Weight/Reps Weight/Reps Weight/Reps Set 1 15 reps / / / / Set 2 (Drop) 10 reps / / / / ABDOMINAL CRUNCH 35-40 REVERSE CRUNCH 20-25 FLUTTER KICKS 35-50 Goals: Perform low-repetition sets with heavier weights than you've been using (This will rapidly improve your strength). Do longer cardiovascular intervals. Improve shoulder-joint integrity to help keep yourself injury-free. 22 Prepare for Airborne School WORKOUT A EXERCISE WEEK 1 WEEK 2 WEEK 3 WEEK 4 Jump Squat Weight/Reps Weight/Reps Weight/Reps Weight/Reps Set 1 12-15 / / / / Set 2 12-15 / / / / Set 3 12-15 / / / / Leg Curls Weight/Reps Weight/ Reps Weight/Reps Weight/Reps Set 1 12-15 / / / / Set 2 12-15 / / / / Set 3 12-15 / / / / Dumbell Step-ups Weight/Reps Weight/Reps Weight/ Reps Weight/Reps Set 1 12-15 / / / / Set 2 12-15 / / / / Set 3 12-15 / / / / Standing Calf Raises Weight/Reps Weight/Reps Weight/Reps Weight/ Reps Set 1 12-15 / / / / Set 2 12-15 / / / / Set 3 12-15 / / / / ABDOMINAL Sit-ups 50-100 Crunches 50-100 Flutter Kicks 25-50 * Practice jump squats with feet and knees together. Reduce the rest time between work sets to fatigue muscles and stimulate muscle growth. 23 Prepare for Airborne School WORKOUT B EXERCISE WEEK 1 WEEK 2 WEEK 3 WEEK 4 Pull-ups Weight/Reps Weight/Reps Weight/Reps Weight/Reps Set 1 12-15 / / / / Set 2 12-15 / / / / Set 3 12-15 / / / / Reverse Close-grip Lat Pull-downs Using Rope Weight/Reps Weight/Reps Weight/Reps Weight/Reps Set 1 12-15 / / / / Set 2 12-15 / / / / Set 3 12-15 / / / / Deadlift Weight/ Reps Weight/Reps Weight/Reps Weight/Reps Set 1 12-15 / / / / Set 2 12-15 / / / / Set 3 12-15 / / / / Push-ups (Regular) Weight/Reps Weight/ Reps Weight/Reps Weight/Reps Set 1 25-50 / / / / Set 2 25-50 / / / /

Set 3 25-50 / / / / Push-ups (Close) Weight/Reps Weight/Reps Weight/ Reps Weight/Reps Set 1 25-50 / / / / Set 2 25-50 / / / / Set 3 25-50 / / / / Front Raises Weight/Reps Weight/Reps Weight/Reps Weight/Reps Set 1 12-15 / / / / Set 2 12-15 / / / / Set 3 12-15 / / / / ABDOMINAL Crunches 50-100 Reverse Crunches 25-50 Flutter Kicks 25-50 For push-ups and pull-ups adjust repetitions to ability. Do negative repetitions with assistance to achieve muscle failure. Rest 2 minutes between sets 24 Prepare for NALC/Air-Assault School WORKOUT A EXERCISE WEEK 1 WEEK 2 WEEK 3 WEEK 4 OBSTACLE COURSE OR CIRCUIT The ideal Obstacle Course would replicate what is found at Air-Assault School. If this is not available, develop a Circuit that includes a rope climb and 6 foot wall at a minimum. Run a minimum of 30 seconds between obstacles. GUERILLA CIRCUIT Conduct each exercise for 20-40 seconds with no rest between All Fours Run 20-40 sec 20-40 sec 20-40 sec 20-40 sec Broad Jump 20-40 sec 20-40 sec 20-40 sec 20-40 sec Crab Walk 20-40 sec 20-40 sec 20-40 sec 20-40 sec Jump Squat 12-15 Reps 12-15 Reps 12-15 Reps 12-15 Reps AGILITY EXERCISES Hour Glass Drill Tree Line Shuffle Drill Ski Hops Star Drill ABDOMINAL SIT-UPS 50-100 SIDE RAISE (Left) 15-25 SIDE RAISE (Right) 15-25 *Run the Obstacle Course or Circuit at least twice. Work up to doing 3 sets (warm-up, moderate and full speed). Rest 2-5 minutes between sets 25 Prepare for NALC & Air-Assault School WORKOUT B EXERCISE WEEK 1 WEEK 2 WEEK 3 WEEK 4 BENCH PRESS Weight/Reps Weight/ Reps Weight/Reps Weight/Reps Flat 5-8 Reps / / / / Incline 5-8 Reps / / / / Decline 5-8 Reps / / / / Dumbbell Shoulder Press Weight/Reps Weight/ Reps Weight/Reps Weight/Reps Work Set 1 5-8 Reps / / / / Work Set 2 5-8 Reps / / / / Work Set 3 5-8 Reps / / / / BICEPS CURL Weight/Reps Weight/Reps Weight/Reps Weight/Reps Work Set 1 5-8 Reps / / / / Work Set 2 5-8 Reps / / / / Work Set 3 / / / / TRICEPS PUSHDOWN Weight/ Reps Weight/Reps Weight/Reps Weight/Reps Work Set 1 5-8 Reps / / / / Work Set 2 5-8 Reps / / / / Work Set 3 5-8 Reps / / / / MACHINE ROW Weight/Reps Weight/Reps Weight/Reps Weight/Reps Work Set 1 5-8 Reps / / / / Work Set 2 5-8 Reps / / / / Work Set 3 5-8 Reps / / / / PULL-UPS Weight/Reps Weight/Reps Weight/Reps Weight/Reps Wide 8-10 Reps / / / / Wrist-out 8-10 Reps / / / / Wrist-in 8-10 Reps / / / / PUSH-UPS Weight/Reps Weight/Reps Weight/Reps Weight/Reps Wide 25-50 Reps / / / / Regular 25-50 Reps / / / / Close 25-50 Reps / / / / ABDOMINAL ELEVATED SIT-UPS 50-100 INCLINE KNEE-UP 25-50 CYCLING TWIST 25-50 26 Training Log Exercise Date Date Date Date Date

Date Date Date Wt/Reps Wt/Reps Wt/Reps Wt/Reps Wt/Reps Wt/Reps Wt/Reps Wt/Reps /

Cardiovascular

____

____

____

27 Resistance Exercises LEGS Quadriceps Front Barbell Squat Preparation From a rack with barbell upper chest height, position bar on front of the shoulders. Cross arms and place hands on top of barbell with upper arms parallel to floor. Dismount bar from rack. Can also be performed on the Smith machine. Execution Descend until thighs are just past parallel. Extend knees and hips until legs are straight. Return and repeat. Comments Keep head forward, back straight and feet flat on the floor; equal distribution of weight through fore foot and heel. Barbell Squat Preparation From a rack with barbell upper chest height, position bar on the back of the shoulders and grasp barbell to sides. Dismount bar from rack. Can also be performed on a squat machine, Smith machine, or with dumbbells. Execution Descend until thighs are just past parallel to floor. Extend knees and hips until legs are straight. Return and repeat.Comments Keep head forward, back straight and feet flat on the floor; equal distribution of weight throughout forefoot and heel. Jump Squat Preparation Assume the squat position on a flat surface. You need squat no further than parallel to the ground. Execution Jump vertically as high as you can and land in the start position. Repeat. Hack Squat Preparation 28 Position barbell just behind legs. With feet flat on floor, squat down and grasp barbell from behind with an overhand grip. Can also be performed on a hack squat machine or Smith machine. Execution Lift bar by extending hips and knees to full extension. Descend until thighs are close to parallel to floor. Repeat. Comments Throughout lift keep hips low, shoulders high, arms and back straight. Lunge Preparation From a rack with barbell upper chest height, position bar on the back of the shoulders and grasp barbell to sides. Dismount bar from rack. Can also be performed with dumbbells. Execution Lunge forward with first leg. Land on heal then forefoot. Lower body by flexing knee and hip of

front leg until knee of rear leg is almost in contact with floor. Return to original standing position by forcibly extending the hip and knee of the forward leg. Repeat by alternating lunge with opposite leg. Comments Keep torso upright during lunge. Rear Lunge Preparation From a rack with barbell upper chest height, position bar on the back of the shoulders and grasp barbell to sides. Dismount bar from rack. Can also be performed with dumbbells. Execution Extend one leg back on forefoot. Lower body on other leg by flexing knee and hip of front leg until knee of rear leg is almost in contact with floor. Return to original standing position by extending the hip and knee of the forward leg. Repeat by alternating lunge with opposite leg. Comments Keep torso upright during lunge; flexible hip flexors are important. A long lunge emphasizes the Gluteus Maximus; a short lunge emphasizes Quadriceps. Step-up Preparation Stand facing the side of a bench. Position bar on the back of the shoulders or grasp barbell to sides. Execution Place foot of first leg on bench. Stand on bench by extending the hip and knee of the first leg and place the foot of second leg on bench. Step down with second leg by flexing the hip and knee of first leg. Return to original standing position by placing foot of first leg to floor. Repeat first step with opposite leg alternating first steps between legs. Comments 29 Keep torso upright during exercise. Stepping a distance from the bench emphasizes the Gluteus Maximus; stepping close to the bench emphasizes Quadriceps. 45° Leg Press Preparation Sit on machine with back on padded support. Place feet on platform. Extend hips and knees. Release dock lever and grasp handles to sides. Execution Lower platform by flexing hips and knees until hips are completely flexed. Return by extending knees and hips. Repeat. Comments Adjust safety brace and back support to accommodate near full range of motion without forcing hips to bend at waist. Leg Extension Preparation Sit on apparatus with back against padded back support. Place front of lower leg under padded lever. Position knee articulation at same axis as lever fulcrum. Grasp handles to sides for support. Execution Move lever forward by extending knees until leg are straight. Return lever to original position by bending knees. Repeat. Comments Stabilizers are used during heavy resistances to prevent body rising off of seat. Seated Leg Press Preparation Sit on machine with back on padded support. Place feet on platform. Grasp handles to sides. Execution Push platform away by extending knees and hips. Return until hips are completely flexed. Repeat. Comments Adjust seat and back support to accommodate near full range of motion without forcing hips to bend at waist. Hamstrings Good-morning Preparation Position barbell on back of shoulders and grasp bar to sides. Execution Bend hips to lower torso forward until parallel to the floor. Raise torso until hips are extended. Repeat. Comments Throughout lift keep back and knees straight 30 Straight-leg Deadlift Preparation Stand with a shoulder width or narrower stance. Grasp barbell with a shoulder width mixed grip or slightly wider; or hold dumbbells at side. Execution With knees straight, lower bar by bending hips until hamstrings are tight, or just before lower back bends. Lift the bar by extending hips until straight. Pull shoulders back at top of lift if rounded. Repeat. Comments Throughout lift keep arms, knees, and back straight. Lying Leg Curl Machine Preparation Facing bench, stand between bench and lever pads. Lie prone on bench with knees just beyond edge of bench and lower legs under lever pads. Grasp handles. Execution Raise lever pads to back of thighs by flexing knees. Lower lever pads until knees are straight. Repeat. Comments Keep torso on bench to reduce hyperextension of the lower back. Most machines are angled at the users hip to position the hamstring in a more favorable mechanical position. Seated Leg Curl Machine Preparation Sit on apparatus with back against padded back support. Place back of lower leg on top of padded lever. Secure lap pad against thigh just above knees. Grasp handles on lap support. Execution Pull lever to back of thighs by flexing knees. Return lever until knees are straight. Repeat. Standing Leg Curl Machine Preparation Stand in machine with one or both legs against pads dependent upon design. Stand foot of resting leg on elevated platform. Position exercising leg: lower leg against lever pad and knee just below thigh pad. Bend over by bending hips and grasp handles for support if available. Execution Pull lever up to back of thigh by flexing knee. Return lever until knee is straight. Repeat. Continue with opposite leg. Comments If hips are not significantly bent, hip flexors act as antagonist stabilizers. Thigh Adduction - Cable Preparation Stand in front of low pulley facing to one side. Attach cable cuff to near ankle. Step out away from the stack with a wide stance and grasp ballet bar. Stand on far foot and allow near leg to be Pulled toward low pulley. 31 Execution Move near leg just in front of far leg by abduction the hip. Return and repeat. Turn around and continue with opposite leg. Seated Thigh Adduction Machine Preparation Sit in machine with heels on bars. Pull in on lever to position legs apart. Release lever into position and grasp bars to sides. Execution Move legs toward one another by adduction of the hip. Return and repeat. Seated Thigh Abduction Machine Preparation Sit in machine with heels on bars. Pull in on lever to position legs together. release lever into position and grasp bars to sides. Execution Move legs away from one another by abduction of the hip. Return and repeat. Calves Standing Calf Raise Preparation Set barbell on power rack upper chest height with calf block under barbell. Position back of shoulders under barbell with both hands to sides. Position toes and balls of feet on calf block with arches and heels extending off. Lean barbell against rack and raise from supports by extending knees and hips. Support barbell against verticals with both hands to sides. Can be done on the leg press machine, with dumbbells, standing one-legged, donkey machine, seated calf machine, and standing calf machine. Execution Raise heels by extending ankles as high as possible. Lower heels by bending ankles until calves are stretched. Repeat. Comments Keep knees straight throughout exercise or bend knees slightly only during stretch. Back Bent-over Row Preparation Bend knees slightly and bend over bar with back straight. Grasp bar with a wide overhand grip. Can also be performed on machine. Execution Pull bar to upper waist. Return until arms are extended and shoulders are stretched forward. Repeat. Bent-over Row w/Dumbbells Preparation 32 Kneel over side of bench with arm and leg to side. Grasp dumbbell. Execution Pull dumbbell to side until upper arm is just beyond horizontal or height of back. Return until arm is extended and shoulder is stretched forward. Repeat. Continue with opposite arm. Comments Allow scapula to articulate but do not rotate torso in an effort to throw weight up. Bent Knee Good-morning Preparation Position barbell on back of shoulders and grasp bar to sides. Execution Bend hips to lower torso forward until parallel to the floor. Bend the knees slightly during the decent. Raise torso until hips are extended. Repeat. Comments Target muscle is exercised isometrically. Throughout lift keep back straight. Quadriceps can be kept bent throughout movement. Deadlift Preparation With feet flat beneath bar squat down and grasp bar with a shoulder width or slightly wider over hand or mixed grip. May use dumbbells also. Execution Lift bar by extending hips and knees to full extension. Pull shoulders back at top of lift if rounded. Return and repeat. Comments Target muscle is exercised isometrically. Throughout lift keep hips low, shoulders high, arms and back straight. Keep bar close to body to improve mechanical leverage. Stiff-leg Deadlift Preparation Stand with a shoulder width or narrower stance on an 8" platform with feet flat beneath bar. Bend over and grasp barbell with a shoulder width or slightly wider overhand or mixed grip. May use dumbbells also. Execution With knees bent, lift the bar by extending at hips until standing upright. Pull shoulders back at top of lift if rounded. Extend knees at top if desired. Lower bar to the top of the feet by bending hips. Bend the knees slightly during the decent and keep waist straight, flexing only slightly at the bottom. Repeat. Comments Lower back may bend slightly during full hip flexion. Target muscle is exercised isometrically if lower back does not bend. Throughout lift keep arms and back straight. Quadriceps can be kept bent throughout movement. Shrug Preparation Stand holding barbell with a overhand or mixed grip; shoulder width or slightly wider. May use dumbbells, cable or machine also. 33 Execution Elevate shoulders as high as possible. Lower and repeat. Comments Since this movement becomes more difficult as full shoulder elevation is achieved, a height criteria for shoulder elevation may be needed. For example, raising the shoulders until the slope of the shoulders become horizontal may be considered adequate depending upon individual body structure. Lying Row Preparation Lie chest down on elevated bench. Grasp dumbbells below. Execution Pull dumbbells to sides until upper arm is just beyond horizontal or height of back. Return until arms are extended and shoulders are stretched forward. Repeat. Comments Bench should be high enough to allow shoulders to stretch forward without dumbbells hitting floor. Back Extension Machine Preparation Sit in machine with back against padded lever. Push hips back against back of seat by pushing feet against platform. Arch back in "C" shape. Execution Extend spine until fully hyperextended. Return and repeat. Comments To avoid hip movement, push hips back into seat by pushing feet into platform throughout exercise. Position foot platform so a small space remains between edge of seat and back of lower thigh. Use seat belt if it becomes difficult to stabilize hips. Hyper-extension bench Preparation Position thighs prone on padding. Hook heels on platform lip or under padded brace. Hold weight to chest or behind neck. Execution Lower body by bending waist until fully flexed. Raise, or extend waist until torso is parallel to legs. Repeat. Comments Although articulation of the waist is emphasized, some hip extension may accommodate movement. If weight is positioned behind head, neck extensors act as stabilizers Pullover Machine Preparation Adjust seat height so lever is near shoulder axis. Sit on machine and Push foot lever. Place elbows in pads and grasp bar from behind. Release foot lever and place feet on platform or to sides. Execution 34 Pull over until elbows are to sides. Return until shoulder is fully flexed, or upper arm is parallel to torso. Repeat. Comments When finished Push foot lever before releasing arm from lever. Release foot lever after releasing arm from lever. One Arm High Row Preparation Sit on platform or bench with knees bent. Grasp cable stirrup with one hand. Straighten lower back and position knees with a slight bend. Allow shoulder with stirrup to be pulled forward with a slight twist through waist. Also done on machine. Execution Pull cable attachment to side, slightly twisting through waist. Pull shoulders back and push chest forward during contraction. Return until arm is extended and shoulder is stretched forward. Repeat. Comments It is optional to bend the lower back forward during the stretch and pull it upright during contraction. In which case, the Erector Spinae becomes a synergist muscle. One Arm Row Preparation Sit on platform or bench with knees bent. Grasp cable stirrup with one hand. Straighten lower back and position knees with a slight bend. Allow shoulder with stirrup to be pulled foward with a slight twist through waist. Also done on machine. Execution Pull cable attachment to side, slightly twisting through waist. Pull shoulders back and push chest forward during contraction. Return until arm is extended and shoulder is stretched forward. Repeat. Comments It is optional to bend the lower back forward during the stretch and pull it upright during contraction. In which case, the Erector Spinae becomes a synergist muscle. Seated High Row Preparation Sit on platform with knees bent and grasp cable attachment. Straighten lower back and position knees with a slight bend. Also done on machine. Execution Pull cable attachment to waist. Pull shoulders back and push chest forward during contraction. Return until arms are extended and shoulders are stretched forward. Repeat. Comments It is optional to bend the lower back forward during the stretch and pull it upright during contraction. In which case, the Erector Spinae becomes a Synergists muscle. Seated Row Preparation Sit on platform with knees bent and grasp cable attachment. Straighten lower back and position knees with a slight bend. Also done on machine. Execution 35 Pull cable attachment to waist. Pull shoulders back and push chest forward during contraction. Return until arms are extended and shoulders are stretched forward. Repeat. Comments It is optional to bend the lower back forward during the stretch and pull it upright during contraction. Close Grip Pull-down Preparation Grasp parallel cable attachment. Sit with thighs under supports. Also done on machine. Execution Pull down cable attachment to upper chest. Return until arms and shoulders are fully extended. Repeat. Front Pull-down Preparation Grasp cable bar with a wide grip. Sit with thighs under supports. Also done on machine. Execution Pull down cable bar to upper chest. Return until arms and shoulders are fully extended. Repeat. Rear Pull-down Preparation Grasp cable bar with a wide grip. Sit with thighs under supports. Execution Pull down cable bar behind neck. Return until arms and shoulders are fully extended. Repeat. Underhand Pull-down Preparation Grasp cable bar with a underhand grip. Sit with thighs under supports. Also done on machine. Execution Pull down cable bar to upper chest until elbows are to the sides. Return until arms and shoulders are fully extended. Repeat. Chin-up Preparation Step up and grasp bar with wide overhand grip. Step down onto assistance lever or platform. Also done on machine. Execution Pull body up until the chin is just above the bar. Lower body until arms and shoulders are fully extended. Repeat. Comments If no assisted machine is used, assist as needed by allowing training partner to pull feet up behind legs or push self up with legs on elevation. 36 Close Grip Chin-up Preparation Step up and grasp parallel grips. Step down onto assistance lever or platform. Also done on machine. Execution Pull body up until elbows are to the sides. Lower body until arms and shoulders are fully extended. Repeat. Comments If no assisted machine is used, assist as needed by allowing training partner to pull feet up behind legs or push self up with legs on elevation. Pull-up Preparation Step up and grasp bar with an wide overhand grip. Step down onto assistance lever or platform. Also done on machine. Execution Pull body up until neck reaches the height of the hands. Lower body until arms and shoulders are fully extended. Repeat. Comments If no assisted machine is used, assist as needed by allowing training partner to pull feet up behind legs or push self up with legs on elevation. Rear Pull-up Preparation Step up and grasp bar with an overhand wide grip. Step down onto assistance lever or platform. Execution Pull body up until the bar touches the back of the neck. Lower body until arms and shoulders are fully extended. Repeat. Comments If no assisted machine is used, assist as needed by allowing training partner to pull feet up behind legs or push self up with legs on elevation. Chest Bench Press Preparation Lie supine on bench. Dismount barbell from rack over the upper chest using a wide oblique overhand grip. Can be performed with dumbbells, on smith machine or press machine. Execution Lower weight to upper chest. Press bar until arms are extended. Repeat. Decline Bench Press Preparation 37 Lie supine on decline bench with feet under leg brace. Dismount barbell from rack over the chest using a wide oblique overhand grip. Can be performed with dumbbells, on smith machine or decline bench machine. Execution Lower weight to upper chest. Press bar until arms are extended. Repeat. Incline Bench Press Preparation

Lie supine on incline bench. Dismount barbell from rack over the upper chest using a wide oblique overhand grip. Can be performed with dumbbells, on smith machine or incline bench machine. Execution Lower weight to upper chest. Press bar until arms are extended. Repeat. Incline Shoulder Raise Preparation Lie supine on incline bench. Dismount barbell from rack with a shoulder width overhand grip. Position barbell over the upper chest with elbows extended. Can be performed with dumbbells, on smith machine or incline press machine. Execution Raise shoulders toward bar as high as possible. Lower shoulders to bench and repeat. Chest Dip Machine Preparation Mount a wide dip bar with an oblique grip. Step down onto assistance lever. Can also be performed on parallel bars, with or without weight. Execution Push body up with elbows away from body and hips slightly bent. Lower body until chest is slightly stretched. Repeat. Lying Fly Preparation Grasp two opposing high pulley dumbbell attachments. Lie supine on bench, in the middle and perpendicular to both pulleys. Slightly bend elbows and internally rotate shoulders so elbows are back. Can also be performed on lying fly machine. Execution Bring cable attachments together in a hugging motion with elbows in a fixed position and shoulders internally rotated so elbows are to the sides. Return to starting position until chests muscle are stretched. Repeat. Cable Crossover Preparation Grasp two opposing high pulley dumbbell attachments. Stand in the middle and perpendicular to both pulleys. Bend hips, knees and elbows slightly. Internally rotate shoulders so elbows are back initially. Execution 38 Bring cable attachments together in a hugging motion with elbows in a fixed position and shoulders internally rotated so elbows are to the sides. Return to starting position until chest muscles are stretched. Repeat. Pullover Preparation Lie upper back perpendicular on bench. Flex hips slightly. Grasp one dumbbell from behind or from side with both hands under inner plate of dumbbell. Position over chest and fix elbows 15° to 30° throughout exercise. Execution Lower dumbbell over and beyond head until upper arm is parallel to torso. Return and repeat. Pec Deck Fly Preparation Sit in machine with back on pad. If available, push foot lever until padded lever moves forward. Place forearms on padded lever. Position upper arms approximately parallel. Release foot lever. Execution Push levers together. Return until chest muscles are stretched. Repeat. Shoulders Behind Neck Press Preparation Grasp barbell with overhand grip from rack or clean from floor. Position bar behind neck. Can be done on machine or using dumbbells. Execution Press bar until arms are extended overhead. Return behind neck and repeat. Front Raise Preparation Grasp barbell with overhand grip. Can be done on machine or using dumbbells. Execution Raise barbell with elbows fixed in a 10° to 30° angle throughout until upper arm is parallel to the floor. Lower and repeat Military Press Preparation Grasp barbell from rack or clean barbell from floor with overhand grip, slightly wider than shoulder width. Position bar in front of neck. Can also be done on machine or using dumbbells. Execution Press bar until arms are extended overhead. Lower to front of neck and repeat Upright Row Preparation 39 Grasp bar with shoulder width or slightly narrower overhand grip. Can be done on machine or using dumbbells. Execution Pull bar to neck with elbows leading. Allow wrists to flex as bar rises. Lower and repeat. Lateral Raise Preparation Grasp stirrup cable attachment. Stand facing with side of resting arm toward low pulley. Grasp ballet bar if available. Can be done using dumbbells, seated, or standing. Execution With elbow slightly bent, raise arm to side away from low Pulley until elbow is shoulder height. Lower and repeat. Lying Rear Lateral Raise Preparation Lie chest down on elevated bench. Grasp dumbbells or cable attachment below to each side. Execution Raise upper arms to sides until shoulder height. Maintain upper arms perpendicular to torso and a fixed elbow position (10° to 30° angle) throughout exercise. Maintain height of elbows above wrists by raising "pinkie" side up. Lower and repeat. Comments Bench should be high enough to prevent dumbbells from hitting floor. Arms Triceps Triceps Dip Preparation Mount a shoulder width dip bar. Step down onto assistance lever if needed. Execution Push body up with elbows close to body and hips straight. Lower body until shoulders are slightly stretched. Repeat. Close Grip Bench Press Preparation Lie on bench and grasp barbell from rack with a close grip. Execution Lower weight to chest with elbows close to body. Return and repeat. Variation Can be done with cables or using dumbbells. Lying Triceps Extension Preparation 40 Lie on bench with a narrow overhand grip on the barbell. Position barbell over the forehead with arms extended. Execution Lower the bar by bending the elbow. As the bar nears the head move the elbows slightly back just enough to allow the bar to clear around the curvature of the head. Extend the arm. As the bar clears the head reposition the elbows to its former position until the arm is fully extended. Repeat. Comments With the arms fully extended, the bar can be brought back over the upper chest and the shoulders can be internally rotated between repetitions as needed to allow for a relative release of tension in the muscles. Variation Can be done with cable or using dumbbell. Triceps Extension Preparation Position barbell overhead with a narrow overhand grip. Can be done on machine or using dumbbells. Execution Lower forearm behind upper arm with elbows remaining overhead. Extend forearm overhead. Lower and repeat. Comments Let the barbell pull the arm back to maintain full shoulder flexion. Pushdown Preparation Grasp cable attachment with overhand grip. Position elbow to side. Execution Extend arm down. Return until forearm is close to upper arm. Repeat. Comments The elbow can travel up a few inches at the top of the motion. Step close to cable to provide resistance at the top of the motion. Kickback Preparation Kneel over bench with arm supporting body. Grasp dumbbell. Position upper arm parallel to floor. Can also be done using cables. Execution Extend arm until it is straight. Return and repeat. Continue with opposite arm. Comments For greater range of motion, upper arm can be positioned with elbow slightly higher than shoulder. Bench Dip Preparation Place weight on lap. Place hands on the edge of a bench, feet on adjacent bench. Execution Lower body until full stretch or rear end touches floor. Raise body and repeat. 41 Biceps Curl Preparation Grasp bar with a shoulder width under hand grip. Can be done on machine, with cables, or using dumbbells. Execution With the elbows to the side, raise the bar until forearms are vertical. Lower until the arms are fully extended. Repeat. Comments When the elbow is fully flexed, the elbow should only travel forward a few inches allowing the forearm to be no more than perpendicular to the floor to allow for a relative release of tension in the muscles between repetitions. Incline Curl Preparation Sit back on a 45-60 degree incline bench. With arms hanging down straight, position two dumbbells with palms facing in. Execution With elbows back to the sides, raise one dumbbell and rotate forearm until forearm is vertical to the floor and the palm faces the shoulder. Lower to original position and repeat with alternative arm. Comments The biceps may be exercised alternating (as described), simultaneous, or in a simultaneous-alternating fashion. When the elbow is fully flexed, the elbow should only travel forward a few inches allowing the forearm to be no more than perpendicular to the floor to allow for a relative release of tension in the muscles between repetitions. Preacher Curl Preparation Sit on preacher bench placing back of arms on pad. The seat should be adjusted to allow the arm pit to rest near the top of the pad. Grasp curl bar with shoulder width underhand grip. Can be done on machine or using dumbbells. Execution Raise the bar until forearms are perpendicular to floor with the back of the upper arm remaining on the pad. Lower the barbell until arm is fully extended. Repeat. Concentration Curl Preparation Sit on bench. Grasp dumbbell between feet. Place back of upper arm to inner thigh. Lean into leg to raise elbow slightly. Execution Raise dumbbell to front of shoulder. Lower dumbbell until arm is fully extended. Repeat. 42 Forearms Reverse Curl Preparation Grasp bar with a shoulder width over hand grip. Can be done on machine or using dumbbells. Execution With the elbows to the side, raise the bar until forearms are vertical. Lower until the arms are fully extended. Repeat. Comments When the elbow is fully flexed, the elbow should only travel forward a few inches allowing the forearm to be no more than perpendicular to the floor to allow for a relative release of tension in the muscles between repetitions. Reverse Preacher Curl Preparation Sit on preacher bench placing back of arms on pad. The seat should be adjusted to allow the arm pit to rest near the top of the pad. Grasp curl bar with shoulder width overhand grip. Can be done on machine or using dumbbells. Execution Raise the bar until forearms are perpendicular to floor with the back of the upper arm remaining on the pad. Lower the barbell until arm is fully extended. Repeat. Hammer Curl Preparation Position two dumbbells to sides, palms facing in, arms straight. Execution With elbows to the sides, raise one dumbbell until forearm is vertical to the floor and the thumb faces the shoulder. Lower to original position and repeat with alternative arm. Comments The biceps may be exercised alternating (as described), simultaneous, or in a simultaneous-alternating fashion. When the elbow is fully flexed, the elbow should only travel forward a few inches allowing the forearm to be no more than perpendicular to the floor to allow for a relative release of tension in the muscles between repetitions. Wrist Curl Preparation Sit and grasp bar with narrow to shoulder width underhand grip. Rest forearms on thighs with wrists just beyond knees. Can be done on machine or using dumbbells. Execution Allow the barbell to roll out of the palms down to the fingers. Grip barbell back up and flex wrists. Lower and repeat. Reverse Wrist Curl Preparation Sit and grasp bar with narrow to shoulder width overhand grip. Rest forearms on thighs with wrists just beyond knees. Can be done on machine or using dumbbells. 43 Execution Hyperextend wrist and return until wrist are fully flexed. Repeat. Abdominal Inline Sit-up Preparation Sit on apparatus with lower leg secured under padded bar. Hold weight to front of chest or behind neck or use no weight. Execution Lower body back until hips are almost extended. Raise body by flexing hips until torso is upright. Repeat. Comments Exercise can be performed without added weight until more resistance is needed. Raise incline to increase resistance. Hanging Leg Raise Preparation Place weight between ankles or use no weight. Grasp and hang from high bar. Execution Raise legs by flexing hips and knees until thighs are just pass parallel to floor. Return until hips and knees are extended. Repeat. Comments Exercise can be performed without added weight until more resistance is needed. Knees may be kept extended throughout leg raise to increase intensity. Incline Leg Raise Preparation Sit on incline board. Place weight between ankles or use no weight. Lie supine on incline board with torso elevated. Grasp feet hooks or sides of board for support. Execution Raise legs by flexing hips and knees until thighs are just past perpendicular to torso. Return until hips and knees are extended. Repeat. Comments Exercise can be performed without added weight until more resistance is needed. Elevate incline to increase resistance. Knees may be kept extended throughout leg raise to increase intensity. Leg Raise Preparation Sit on end of bench. Place weight between ankles, hook feet to cable attachment, or use no weight. Lie supine on bench with torso elevated. Grasp bench for support. Execution 44 Raise legs by flexing hips and knees until thighs are just past perpendicular to torso. Return until hips and knees are extended. Repeat. Comments Exercise can be performed without added weight until more resistance is needed. Knees may be kept extended throughout leg raise to increase intensity. Roman Chair Sit-up Preparation Sit on apparatus with lower leg secured under padded bar. Hold weight to front of chest or behind neck or use no weight. Execution Lower body back until hips are almost extended. Raise body by flexing hips until torso is upright. Repeat. Comments Exercise can be performed without added weight until more resistance is needed. Rectus Abdominis and Obliques only contract dynamically if actual waist flexion occurs. With no waist flexion, Rectus Abdominis and External Oblique will only act to stabilize the pelvis and waist during hip flexion. Vertical Leg Raise Preparation Place weight between ankles or use no weight. Position body on padded parallel bars with hands on handles, back on vertical pad, and body weight supported on forearms. Execution Raise legs by flexing hips and knees until thighs are just pass parallel to floor. Return until hips and knees are extended. Repeat. Comments Exercise can be performed without added weight until more resistance is needed. Knees may be kept extended throughout leg raise to increase intensity. Kneeling Crunch Preparation Kneel below a high pulley. Grasp cable rope attachment and place wrists against the head. Flex hips slightly and allow the weight to hyperextend the lower back. Execution With the hips stationary, flex the waist so the elbows travel toward the middle of the thighs. Return and repeat. Variation Can be done on machine. Seated Crunch Preparation Seat with back support away from a medium high Pulley. Grasp cable rope attachment with both hands and place securely over the both shoulders. Allow the weight to hyperextend the lower back slightly. Execution 45 With the hips stationary, flex the waist so the elbows travel toward the hips. Return and repeat. Can be done on machine. Incline Crunch Preparation Hook feet under padding and lie supine on incline bench with hips bent. Hold plate behind neck or on chest with both hands or use no weight. Execution Flex waist to raise upper torso from bench. Return until the back of the shoulders contact the padded incline board. Repeat. Comments Exercise can be performed without added weight until more resistance is needed. Elevate incline to increase resistance. Hip and knee flexors may be involved as stabilizers if incline is steep and no calf support is used. Incline Hip Raise Preparation Sit on incline board. Place weight between ankles or use no weight. Lie supine on incline board with torso elevated. Grasp feet hooks or sides of board by head for support. Execution Raise legs by flexing hips while flexing knees until hips are fully flexed. Continue to raise knees toward shoulders by flexing waist, raising hips from board. Return until waist, hips and knees are extended. Repeat. Comments Exercise can be performed without added weight until more resistance is needed. Elevate incline to increase resistance. When raising hips, keep knees fully flexed as not to throw weight of lower legs over head. Incline Twisting Crunch Preparation Hook feet under padding and lie supine on incline bench with hips bent. Hold plate behind neck or on chest with both hands or use no weight. Execution Flex and twist waist to raise upper torso from bench to one side. Return until the back of the shoulders contact the padded incline board. Repeat to the opposite side alternating twists. Comments Exercise can be performed without added weight until more resistance is needed. Elevate incline to increase resistance. Hip and knee flexors may be involved as stabilizers if incline is steep and no calf support is used. Incline Twisting Sit-up Preparation 46 Hook feet under padding and lie supine on incline bench with hips bent. Hold plate behind neck or on chest with both hands. Execution Flex and twist the waist to one direction while raising the torso from bench by bending hips. Return until the back of the shoulders contact the padded incline board. Repeat to the opposite side alternating twists. Comments Pectineus, Adductor Longus, and Brevis do not assist in hip flexion since hips are already initially bent. Knee flexors may be involved as stabilizers if incline is steep and no calf support is used. Twisting Crunch Preparation Lie supine on bench with head hanging off and knees and hips bent. Hold plate behind neck or on chest with both hands. Execution Flex and twist waist to raise upper torso from bench to one side. Return until the back of the shoulders contact the padded board. Repeat to the opposite side alternating twists. Side Bend Preparation With side to low Pulley, grasp dumbbell cable with near arm. Stand with arm straight. Execution Bend waist to opposite side of cable. Lower and repeat. Turn around and continue with opposite side. Can also be done with dumbbell. Crunch Circuit Preparation Lie flat on your back with your legs straight and raised so that the bottom of your feet are pointed towards the sky Execution Crunch for set number of repetitions then without resting. Bend knees so that legs are at 90 , continue to crunch for set number of repetitions, then without resting lower bent legs to the left 45 from the floor, continue to crunch for set number of repetitions, then without resting lower legs to the right 45 from the floor, continue to crunch for set number of repetitions, then without resting repeat first two steps. Cycling Twist Preparation Lie flat on the ground with your legs fully extended to the front 6 inches off the ground and your upper body raised at a 30 degree angle off the ground. Your hands are joined together at the waist. Execution 47 On alternating movements you will turn your body to one side while bringing the opposite side knee toward your chest. Without allowing your feet to touch the ground, twist your body alternating to the other side. Your legs will alternate with your body twist in a similar movement to cycling. Your hands remain joined the entire time. Flutter Kicks Preparation Lie on your back and place your hands under your buttocks for support. Lift your head, just enough to see your feet and then lift both legs 6 inches off the ground. Execution Lift one leg at least 25 degrees then alternate your legs at a quick tempo. Flexibility Exercises Neck Rotation - Stand with the back straight and feet shoulder width apart. Place the hands on hips. Roll the head slowly to the left, making a complete circle with the path of the head. Reverse direction. See figure Arm and Shoulder Rotation - Stand with the back straight and feet shoulder width apart. Extend the arms outward to shoulder height. Rotate the shoulders forward, making a large circular motion with the arms. Reverse direction. 48 Hip Rotation - Stand with the back straight and feet shoulder width apart. Place the hands on hips. Rotate the hips clockwise while keeping the back straight. Reverse direction. Knee and

Ankle Rotation - Stand with the feet together, and bend at the waist with the knees slightly bent. Place the hands above the knees, and rotate the legs in a clockwise direction. Reverse direction. Neck and Shoulder Stretch - Stand with the feet shoulder width apart and the arms behind the body. Grasp the left wrist with the right hand. Pull the left arm down and to the right. Tilt the head to the right. Hold this position for 10 to 15 seconds. Repeat the action with the right wrist, pulling the right arm down and to the left. Tilt the head to the left. Abdominal Stretch - Stand and extend the arms upward and over the head. Interlace the fingers with palms turned upward. Stretch the arms up and slightly back. Hold this position for 10 to 15 seconds. 49 Chest Stretch - Stand and interlace the fingers behind the back. Lift the arms behind so that they move outward and away from the body. Lean forward from the waist. Hold this position for 10 to 15 seconds. Bend the knees before moving to the upright position. Return to the starting position. Upper-back Stretch - Stand with the arms extended to the front at shoulder height with the fingers interlaced and palms facing outward. Extend the arms and shoulders forward. Hold this position for 10 to 15 seconds. Return to the starting position. Overhead Arm Pull - Stand with the feet shoulder width apart. Raise the right arm, bending the right elbow and touching the right elbow and touching the right hand to the back of the neck. Grab the right elbow with the left hand, and pull to the left. Hold this position for 10 to 15 seconds. Return to the starting position. Do the same stretch, and pull the left elbow with the right hand for 10 to 15 seconds. 50 Thigh Stretch - Stand or lie on the stomach. Bend the left leg up toward the buttocks. Grasp the toes of the left foot with the right hand, and the heel to the left buttock. Extend the left arm to the side for balance. Hold this position for 10 to 15 seconds. Return to the starting position. Switch sides. Hamstring Stretch (Standing) - Stand with the knees slightly bent. Bend forward keeping the head up, and reach toward the toes. Straighten the legs, and hold this position for 10 to 15 seconds. Hamstring Stretch (Seated) - Sit on the ground with both legs straight and extended forward with the feet upright about six inches apart. Put the hands on the ankles or toes. Bend from the hips, keeping the back and head in a comfortable, straight line. Hold this position for 10 to 15 seconds. 51 Groin Stretch (Standing) - Lunge over to the left while keeping the right leg straight, the right foot facing straight ahead and entirely on the floor. Lean over the left leg while stretching the right groin muscles. Hold this position for 10 to 15 seconds. Repeat with the opposite leg. Groin Stretch (Seated) - Sit on the ground with the soles together. Place the hands on or near he feet. Bend forward from the hips, keeping the head up. Hold this position for 10 to 15 seconds. Calf Stretch - Stand straight with the feet together, arms extended downward, elbows locked, palms facing backward, fingers extended and joined, and head and eyes facing front. Move the right foot to the rear about two feet, and place the ball of the foot on the ground. Slowly press the right heel to the ground. Slowly bend the left knee while pushing the hips forward and arching the back slightly. Hold this position for 10 to 15 seconds. Return to the starting position. Repeat with the left foot. Hip and Back Stretch (Seated) – Sit on the ground with the right leg forward and straight. Cross the left leg over the right while sitting erect. Keep the heels of both feet in contact with the ground. Slowly rotate the upper body to the left and look over the left shoulder. Reach across the left leg with the right arm, and push the left leg to your right. Use the left hand for support by placing it on the ground. Hold this position for 10 to 15 seconds. Repeat this stretch for the other side by crossing and turning in the opposite direction. 52 Hip and Back Stretch (Lying Down) - Lie on the back with the arms straight beside the body. Keep the legs straight and the knees and feet together. Bring the left leg straight back toward the head, leaving the right leg in the starting position. Bring the head and arms up. Grab the bent left leg below the knee, and pull it gradually to the chest. Hold this position for 10 to 15 seconds. Gradually return to the starting position. Repeat these motions with the opposite leg. Variation - Pull both knees to the chest. Pull the head up to the knees. Hold for 10 to 15 seconds. Return to the starting position. Agility Exercises All fours run Place your hands in front of you and run using your hands and feet. Broad Jump Jump forward on both feet in a series of broad jumps. Swing the arms vigorously to help with the jumps. Crab Walk Place your hands and feet on the ground, hands behind you and stomach facing the sky. Walk on hands and feet from this position. Hour Glass Drill 53 Mark out a box 10 meters x 10 meters. Start at the front left corner of the box. Run across the front (shoulders square to the front) to the front right corner. Back peddle to the center spot, then out to the back right corner. Run across the back to the back left corner. Run forward to the center spot, then out to the left corner. Three Line Shuffle Drill Mark three parallel lines on the floor, 4 feet apart. Straddle the center line. Begin by shuffling to the far left line, then to the far right, then left, etc. for the allotted time, crossing each line with the foot. Bench Jumps From a standing position, bend your knees slightly and jump to the side (laterally), pushing off with both feet and landing up on a low bench/step. (Beginners may start out without the bench and simply land on the floor.) Come to a full stop, then jump off the other side of the bench and repeat. Ski Hops Mark out lines approximately 3 feet apart and 10 meters in length. Start on one side of the paired lines and jump across to the outside of the other line, progressing down the 10 meters. At the end of the 10 meter, immediately jump across the two lines working backward to the original starting point. Forward; Back. Star Drill Mark out eight points 3 to 5 steps from a center mark, creating a star pattern. Begin rill standing at the center point. Now run out to the first point of the star then back to the center point. Continue to run to each point in the star coming back to the center each time.

CHAPTER TWO

Easy Way to Get Fit

It's another Monday and you're exhausted. You spent the weekend running – running errands, running the kids to activities, running to the service station, running to the grocery store, the home and garden supply store and, well, running yourself ragged. You did everything you set out to do except the one thing you had PROMISED yourself you do — exercise. If you're like most of us you were annoyed when you realize that, once again, you didn't make time for you. Then you felt guilty. After all, your family, friends and colleagues need you. Maybe you will try again next weekend...or the next....or the next.... Sound familiar? You can change that pattern! The first step to Get Fit is to realize this one axiom: You are NOT alone. Researchers have found that 50% of those who start exercise programs quit within the first six months, according to Len Kravitz, Ph.D., program coordinator of exercise science and a researcher at the University of New Mexico in Albuquerque The reason? People are convinced they will fail, even before they start. It doesn't have to be that way! Believe me, I know how you feel. Sure, I am a physical fitness professional and my lifestyle centers on healthy living. But that doesn't mean I don't face the same challenges and roadblocks you do. Kids, work, errands, housework, community events, volunteer work and more —it saps my time, energy and motivation just like it does yours. Let's be honest: none of us have a perfect life, but I found... SMART STEPS lead you to GET FIT and stay that way. You know why exercise is important. Sure, we would all love to gaze into a mirror and see a trim, toned person reflected back. But the real benefit to moving and eating right is the high energy you feel, the strength you exude and the positive attitude you project. Those are the elements that fuel your body and spirit and allow you to work, play, nurture and do all the other things that fill your day. Now I'm not going to pepper you with stories about how weight is linked to disease and may shorten your life span. You know all of that. But I must say two words about it — Tom Hanks. Were you as surprised as many of us were when the 57-year old actor announced he has Type 2 Diabetes? He always seems to exude such health and energy. So how did he develop diabetes? Weight. Remember how he gained and lost weight for movie roles including "A League of Their Own," and "Cast Away?" Tom Hanks thinks his yo-yo weight may have played a role in his diabetes. "The gaining and the losing of weight may have had something to do with [developing diabetes] because you eat so much bad food and you don't exercise when you're heavy," Hanks said at a London press .

No matter how famous or how wealthy people become, everyone struggles to get – and stay fit, even Tom Hanks.

conference, according to "Health" magazine. Now I'm not saying this to scare you. You likely already know what Etie S. Moghissi, M.D., associate clinical professor of medicine at the University of California, Los Angeles and a past vice president of the American Association of Clinical Endocrinologists, said in the same article: "The risk of getting diabetes increases as we gain weight." I'm saying this to tell you that all of us—no matter how wealthy, successful or stable—face the same obstacle to fitness. Now here's the good news — You've already begun to get healthy with..... Step 1: Reading this book. Educating yourself about what works and what doesn't in fitness is the most crucial thing you can do. That's why I wrote this book and that's why reading it is critical to your success. Sure, it seems simple. But that's the secret those selling the big money exercise equipment and fad diets don't tell you. The way to fitness IS simple. And it doesn't require buying their high-priced equipment or special foods. So don't stop now! Keep going to ... Step 2: Walk. Walk around your house. Walk around your yard. Walk around your neighborhood. Do your legs feel tired? What about your feet? Really get in tune with your body and make notes about what feels good and what doesn't. Getting started is the hard part — but you can do it! Step 3: Invest 20 minutes. That's all it will take when you come to my store and let us analyze how you walk, your "gait." Now don't panic. I promise we're not selling you anything you don't need. We just want you to come in for a FREE "gait" analysis. No cost. No obligation. No fear. No pressure.

Think of it this way. When you can't see, don't you go to a vision specialist? When your tooth aches, don't you go see a dentist? So why What's your gait analysis telling you? Everyone usually has one of 3 gaits as illustrated here. However, different shoes and different styles are designed for different gaits. That's why we spend the time to find the shoes that fit your gait. Think of it this way. When you can't see, don't you go to a vision specialist? When your tooth aches, don't you go see a dentist? So why not come to us to find out how to take the pain out of walking and reap the benefits from it and, yes, GET FIT? And unlike the vision specialist and the dentist, we won't charge you for our expertise. Not one penny. Think back to what we discussed about why most fitness programs fail — because exercisers believe they won't be successful. And why is that? You can bet one reason is they start to work out and their feet and legs hurt. No one wants to experience pain. See, when most people start fitness programs, they don't give any thought to their shoes. That can hurt you — literally — because ... to get the most from your work out, you need to make sure the shoe you wear is made for your foot and body and the way it moves. Otherwise your workout is ineffective. And, more important, you risk injury to your legs, feet, back, and core. Only with the help of a trained professional can you choose if you need shoes that provide stability, support or cushion. Come into my store and we'll show you. We'll watch you walk. We'll ask you to jog. Why is that important? When you walk, your feet absorb about two times your body weight. When you run, they may sustain an impact three times your body weight. So choosing the shoes with the right support protects your feet, legs, hips and core, and gives you more energy. Think of it this way—My goal is to fit you in a shoe that is so comfortable that you could play the piano with your toes (Like our aforementioned hero, Tom Hanks, did in the movie 'Big.') Now I bet you're thinking, "Oh this is just a way to get me to spend more money!" I won't kid you. I don't want you to buy the wrong shoes. And if you're selecting shoes based on color and style and bargain prices, chances are those shoes aren't right for you. What do I mean by that? Just that your legs will ache, your feet will be sore and you'll give up on walking, jogging or running almost before you begin. And you may even injure yourself. You'll end up tossing those "bargain" shoes in the back of the closet and abandoning your fitness plan. Consider this: I don't want to sell you the wrong shoes and keep you from pursuing your goals of living healthy and enjoying life. Why is this so important to me? Here's why Step 4: Discover the shoe you need. When you and I work together, you will learn what shoe you need to wear to GET FIT. Now here's my promise: Whether you buy now or at some other time — or never – is up to you. But this step will propel you even closer to success. And it may just change your life. Fan mail like this, from one of my customers, is the reason I can make this promise.

The bottom line is, I want you to come back to my store with your friends. And I want you to tell your family, your friends, your hair stylist, and everyone else that your healthy life started with GET FIT. But let's be clear —I'm not promising that I will get you into shoes at bargain basement prices. But I do promise you that I will get you into the shoe that is designed for your feet, your legs and your body so you can, finally, GET FIT and stay healthy. Of course that's not all you need to GET FIT. The other simple strategies are still built around planning and moderation. WAIT! Has your mind wandered? Are you now thinking about the quickest way to hit your goal? Maybe that diet plan you just saw in the back of the magazine would be the way to go. STOP! You know better. The problem with those "Quick" fitness and diet plans is they just don't work. And no matter what you have heard about the latest and greatest pill, food or equipment, there's only one true way to get and stay healthy, fit, toned and trim. And it's not in a bottle, a special diet, starvation or grueling workouts. I have spent years studying the science behind health and fitness. And I can tell you from experience— not just mine but that of the students and clients with whom I have worked—that science works to make you toned, fit and a calorieburning machine. It all comes down to two things: Moderation and Consistency. That's how you GET FIT. NOW is the time for you to forget all the crazy machines, the unhealthy diets, the promises that go nowhere and use these 5 keys to unlock the healthy you. Key One: Plan. Just like you will come in for gait analysis to ensure you take the pain out of walking and running, you want to plan other parts of your fitness lifestyle. Perhaps one of the most important ways to do that is to write your goals. Sounds crazy but it works. Write down your goals —in a planner, on a calendar, on a piece of paper you hang on your bathroom mirror, and you will succeed!

WARNING! If you're selecting bargain-priced shoes based on color and style, you may wind up paying for it in more ways than one.

Key Two: Buddy Up. Get a work out partner. And no, that's probably not your significant other. Instead, pair with someone whose goals, strength and schedule best compliment yours. Key Three: Practice moderation. We've talked about it. And you've seen it. Maybe you've even lived it. We're talking about people who haven't walked or run in years trying to run a 5K the first day they start exercising. That not only sets you up for failure, but injury. Start slow. Increase gradually. Key Four: Work with a fitness pro. Sure, you may have been an athlete in high school or college, but we're all older now and our bodies have changed. And that brings on new challenges. One thing I've found is that many women who return to exercise complain of knee pain. That's not unusual. Your body needs to become strong again. That's why a fitness professional can help you understand and build hip, core, and leg strength. The pro can also help you devise a cross training plan that will help you reach your goals. Key Five: Nutrition. No, that doesn't mean you need to eat lettuce and celery all day. In fact, you shouldn't. You also shouldn't try all the fancy nutrition bars, diet supplements and energy drinks on the market. Just like everything else, education and moderation is key. There are countless books and diets out there that explain nutrition so I won't dwell on it. I will say, though, that total deprivation, just like gorging, is not the way to GET FIT. Drink water. Eat fruits, veggies and lean meats. And don't overdo anything, even the water. Your Next Step.... Is to call or drop by my store and let us analyze your gait for FREE. Again, I promise we're not going to pressure you to buy. Candidly, we don't need to. I bet once you experience how strong, healthy and yes, pain free, you feel in the proper shoes for your stride, you'll understand why GET FIT will start you on your journey to better health and fitness. Better still listen to what one of my new customers has to say about how GET FIT changed her life: One of my friends convinced me that running would help me lose weight and feel healthy. When I walked in to Get Fit, I was skeptical and thought I would not fit in because everyone was so in shape. Well, I was very wrong. The employees at Get Fit were so motivating and helpful. Without them, I am not sure where I would be. Through the running classes I have met life-long friends and reached goals that I never thought possible. Without the wonderful employees at Get Fit, I would still be an overweight couch potato! But now, because of them, I have my life and health under control. I am down over 50 pounds and about to run my very first half marathon and have nobody to thank but Get Fit!!!! -- Brandi Cota While you're there, talk to us. We're ready to answer your questions and help you GET FIT.

Take the next step ... It may be the most important one of your life! As a reader of this book, you're serious about getting healthy and getting fit – and we want to help. Whether you're just getting started, want to get back into living a healthy lifestyle or you're a lifelong health nut who is looking for others who share your passion, you're invited to stop by our store or visit us online to learn more at fitness first house.

CHAPTER THREE

Intelligent Person's Guide to Fitness

A healthy lifestyle is an intelligent combination of exercise, nutrition and positive mind-set. Being healthy and fit is often a matter of our own choice. If you are smart, you will take an elevator to reach the 10th floor; if you are smarter, you will take the stairs. The choice is yours! Your choice of a lifestyle mainly depends on how you perceive your body. Do you identify yourself with your body? Or, treat it as a sacred tool to achieve something worthwhile in your life? As ancient Sanskrit poet Kalidasa wrote, shariramadyam khalu dharmasadhanam (Our body is the tool to perform our dharma (duty). If you treat your body as a sacred tool, you will not abuse it. Rather, you will train it hard and feed it on right nutrition. On the other hand, if you identify yourself with your body, you will tend to be comfort-loving; you will detest hard work and indulge in immediate sensual gratification e.g., sitting in front of TV for hours and binging on pizza! The choice is always yours! 10 Mantras to Remember Before you undertake an exercise programme, remember these ten Mantras – (i) Human body is a complex machine. Two individuals would not respond alike to the same exercise or nutrition because of their peculiarities of genetics, age, sex, medical history, body composition, Resting Metabolic Rate (RMR)1 , emotional well being, etc. Therefore, you have to experiment with your body and find the best exercise and nutrition solutions that suit you.

(ii) Look around to find 'real' people who are healthy and fit. Study their pattern of exercise, nutrition and lifestyle and see if something can work for you also. You may get many small but useful tips from them, e.g., wearing underwear one size smaller or shoes one size larger than your regular size can make your long runs more comfortable; or, a banana before or during your exercise may provide a wonderful fuel throughout your exercise session. (iii) The subject of health and fitness is quite vast. Therefore, other aspects should also be taken care of. For example, you may never realize that chronic sleep debt or mental stress might be restraining you from reaching your peak performance despite having excellent exercise regimen and balanced diet. (iv) Know the basics of exercise and nutrition, but be bold enough to experiment with what you see around – without any prejudice. Many of the top world sports persons are vegetarian and practice Yoga, Tai chi, meditation to enhance their performance. (v) Mind and body influence each other. Without focus of mind you cannot reach your peak training potential. 'My mind is everything. My muscles are pieces of rubber' – Paavo Nurmi (all time great distance runner, holder of 22 world records.) Similarly, the state of your body also affects your state of mind. Try this next time – when you are depressed – put on your running shoes, run slowly for 40-60 minutes and your depression would vanish! (vi) Give your body its proper place in your overall scheme of things. Don't extol your body beyond what it deserves. A body-centric approach may lead you to disgusting obsession with your body and you may end up taking power performance drugs like steroids. A healthy body with a healthy mind should be our objective. 7 (vii) Don't expect miracles overnight. Beware of all those books, machines and miracle foods claiming to give you muscular body with six-pack abs within a week or month without any workout. Fortunately, there is no alternative to intelligent and hard (and harder) work (outs)! Keep patience. Take no short cuts. Generally, one reaches one's peak potentiality after 40-42 weeks of persistent and scientific training, though benefits of exercise start to appear from the first week itself. (viii) Be an intelligent investor. Invest more time and money for your health and fitness. Take out daily at least half an hour for vigorous exercise. This is the best Life Insurance Policy ever invented! (ix) Never compete with others. Compete against yourself. By competing against others you may get into too much too soon trap and end up injuring yourself – physically, mentally and emotionally! (x) Aim for fitness with health. You must understand that health and fitness are two different things. Physical health can be described as smooth functioning of all our systems including nervous, energy, skeletal, endocrine, cardiovascular systems; it is not merely absence of any disease. Mental and emotional well being is the other important aspect of health. Fitness, on the other hand, is one's ability to meet certain measurable physical standards for a particular job, e.g., fitness for army, college football team, etc. You may be an impressive body builder but in the process if you have overburdened your kidneys with high-protein diet, that is not a fitness with health. An intelligent person will never pursue fitness at the cost of his health. Draw a bigger line Once you have realized the importance of healthy lifestyle, the next challenge is to keep yourself constantly on the track. For this you require a positive approach towards exercise. Sometimes exercise and nutrition is 8 'prescribed' as a complementary preventive, regulatory or curative medicine for certain diseases. Many persons start exercise only after they are detected with some disease, e.g., diabetes or heart disease. They take exercise as a bitter pill. This is not a right approach to start exercise and like most of the New Year resolutions this also will not take you very far. I laugh at the ways suggested sometimes by health magazines and articles in newspapers for fat loss e.g., how to control your cravings for 'good' food. Even Gastric Bypass surgery is suggested! Don't take up exercise 'just to be fit'. Adopt healthy lifestyle as celebration of life. Aim BIG. For example, aim to run half marathon next year. Once you start training for the half marathon, automatically junk foods, late night parties or late morning sleeps will fast lose their attraction for you. Nutritious food and regular training sessions will replace your lethargic routine. Remember, aiming big is the only way to steer clear of small temptations in life. It's for everyone, everywhere The scope of this book has been deliberately kept limited to free hands exercises which can be performed anywhere. You may like to do them with your partner. Once you have mastered the basics of exercise, you may also like to invest in a few sets of free weights. Buy dumb bells, bench, chin up bar. That's all. Do exercise with whatever is available. But do start. Use stairs of hotels, do skipping in the room, do circuit training in your room. A space of 6' x 6' is big enough for exercise. Knowledge is for action Learn the basics of exercise and nutrition. Learn more than the basics. And, apply the knowledge. "Knowing is not enough; we must apply." -Goethe. Maintain a log book to keep record of your daily exercise regimen, nutrition and monitor your progress in fitness and well-being. Experiment with 9 yourself. And see for yourself what really works for you. For example, you may observe after some time that your body requires a little longer recovery period. Or, your body system is not comfortable with dairy products. Finally, set your focus right. Focus on fitness and health, not on the shape or weight of your body. As long as you have steady progress in health and fitness, you should not worry about your shape or weight. Genetically very few persons have been endowed with the potentiality of building a model's physique. However, this should not disappoint you. Look at the top sportspersons in any field of sports to realize this truth. You will find that very few of them have a model's physique, though all of them are supremely fit! If you are constantly worried about your weight, I must tell you that ironically, weighing machine is the most used though most useless equipment in a gym. This issue will be discussed in detail in the chapter on Weight Management. II. BENEFITS OF EXERCISE These are the major benefits of exercise – (i) It delays biological aging. Your aging process is influenced by your genetics, environment and lifestyle. Let me explain that chronological aging is different from biological aging. For instance, all persons born on 05 th February 1966 will inevitably turn 45 on 05th February 2011 (this is chronological age). But not two of these persons will be of the same biological age at any given point of time! Interesting? This is because biological aging is the aging of our biological systems, i.e., cardiovascular, skeletal system, etc. Thus it is quite possible that heart of a trained athlete of 60 may be biologically younger than that of a sedentary person of 30. Next time when someone asks your age, ask him back – chronological or biological one? 10 Regular exercise delays aging process in the following ways – (a) As you age, there is decline in efficiency of your cardiovascular system. By regular exercise, especially aerobic exercise, your VO2 max (V – Volume; O2 – Oxygen; max – Maximum.) improves. VO2 max refers to uptake of maximal oxygen and its utilization by your body. A higher VO2 max means – (a) your heart's capacity to pump blood is increased; (b) your lungs' capacity to fill themselves with larger volume of oxygen is increased; (c) your arteries and blood vessels can deliver more oxygen; (d) your muscles will utilize oxygen more efficiently. The net result of all these will be that you will tire less even at a higher intensity of activity. (b) We lose about 0.2 kg of muscle per year during our 30s and 40s. This process of muscle loss is called sarcopenia. The rate of muscle loss may double up to 0.45 kg per year in people past 50 years2 . Regular exercise, especially strength training, decreases the rate of muscle loss. Strength training contributes to strength gain at any age. (i) It helps to prevent cardiovascular diseases, stroke, type II diabetes, cancer of colon. (ii) Low-intensity endurance training has a lowering effect in cases of high blood pressure. (iii) It helps to increase HDL (High density lipoprotein) and decrease LDL (Low density lipoprotein). Lower LDL and higher HDL means a decreased risk of coronary heart disease. (iv) It reduces total body fat and makes you leaner. (v) It increases bone strength and is helpful in preventing those nasty bathroom hip fractures in advanced age. (vi) It also strengthens cartilage, tendons and ligaments makes them more flexible and thus prevents injury. (vii) It improves immunity against various diseases. (viii) It improves overall strength, endurance, flexibility, agility, motor coordination and balance.

(ix) Regular exercise improves brain power, gives lightness of body, decreases anxiety and depression, makes you confident and enhances the feeling of well-being. It gives you sufficient energy reserve to excel in your day to day life whether at home or at work place. III. PRINCIPLES OF EXERCISE To design an effective exercise programme, certain basic principles of exercise must be followed. These principles are equally important for everyone, whether one is an elite athlete or a common exerciser. The basic principles of exercise are– (i) Regularity – Regularity means that all exercises for cardiovascular endurance, muscle strength and flexibility should be done at least 3-5 times a week at regular intervals. Regularity in exercise promotes better performance by allowing regular load and then adequate rest to exercised muscles. Long gap between two exercise sessions may cause de-conditioning of muscles during which gains in strength, endurance or flexibility, etc. are considerably reduced or lost. Moreover, injuries are frequent results of irregular exercise sessions because de-conditioned muscles are mindlessly subjected to the same (previous) training load despite their decreased strength in the meantime. (ii) Progression – Progression means that there should be gradual increase in intensity and volume of exercise. Increase in intensity means an increase in weight (in weight/resistance training) or an increase in heart rate (in endurance training). Similarly, increase in volume means an increase in number of repetitions (reps)/sets (in weight/resistance training) or an increase in total duration (in endurance training). Stressing your system too much too soon may actually harm you. It may cause overtraining and injury. Therefore, first know your existing baseline fitness level and gradually go on increasing the load. (See the section on Strength Training/Endurance Training for practical 12 guidelines on the rate of progression). It is always advisable to start with 2–3 weeks of gradual conditioning by doing light exercises before you graduate to a full-fledged exercise programme. (iii) Balance – Balance means that an exercise programme must address all components of fitness, viz., endurance, strength, flexibility, speed, agility, etc. (See the section on Components of Fitness). However, there may be specific weightage on a particular component based on one's training goal. For example, a marathon runner may focus more on endurance training while a football player may train mainly in speed, agility and strength. But irrespective of one's training goal, one has to maintain certain basic balance among various components of fitness. Secondly, we have to balance between upper body and lower body as well as between opposite muscles. For example, it is necessary to keep balance between strength of quadriceps and hamstrings or between biceps and triceps to avoid injury. I have noticed many gym goers focusing mainly on exercising their upper body(which can be showed off to others) and ignoring their lower body. This is not a balanced approach. (iv) Variation – Variation means (i) introducing different variations of an exercise and (ii) addressing muscle groups from various angles. If you stick to the same type of exercises for the same muscle groups for a period of time, you are bound to neglect certain other muscle groups in the process. This will result into weakness of unaddressed muscle groups. Variation is also helpful for overall development of a particular muscle group. Therefore, once in a while, add variation to your exercise programme for maximal gain. For example, performing push-ups at various hand-widths (narrow, shoulder-width, wide) or in various positions (inclined, declined, flat) will address the related muscles more widely. Variation also helps us to fight monotony.

v) Overload – By overloading we mean frequently crossing the training threshold while maintaining the right form and technique. You cannot gain any further unless you challenge your body beyond its normal capacity. If you can do 20 push-ups today, overload yourself by doing further two more push ups, then one more, and one more ... till your muscles fail totally. The more you load your system, the greater will be your training gains. If you continue with the same training load over a long period of time, your training gain will decrease due to accommodation of your system to the present load. Therefore, the key to maximal gain is to overload your system. You may overload your system by increasing intensity or volume of the exercise. Here, again, you should avoid 'too much too soon' approach. (vi) Specificity – Specificity means designing an exercise programme for a specific group of muscles/specific component of fitness (see the section on Components of Fitness) for a specific goal. For example, a police officer may have goal of overall fitness, but a weight lifter will train specifically for strength. Similarly, training for a distance runner will be more endurance-focused training. However, one should go for specific training only after a general training on overall fitness. For example, a marathon runner, though specifically training for endurance, also needs strength and flexibility training. There are certain basic exercises which will benefit all the beginners and their overall fitness will improve. It is advisable that you should first do the basic training in strength, endurance and flexibility, and then only go for your goal-specific training. (vii) Recovery — Recovery means allowing your exercised muscles sufficient rest between two sets/exercise sessions. The body repairs and strengthens itself during rest. When you exercise a muscle, the stress of exercise causes (i) muscle tissue breakdown and (ii) muscle glycogen depletion (loss of energy store). Recovery time allows replenishment of energy store and repair of broken down muscle tissues. During rest period muscles grow stronger. Not allowing sufficient 14 recovery time may result in overtraining (see section on Overtraining) which may further cause (i) reduction in performance and (ii) injury. Duration of recovery period may vary from 48 to 72 hours depending on the intensity and volume of training. Alternating hard training day and easy training day is also another way of recovery. This has been discussed in detail in the chapter on Exercise Programme Design. IV. COMPONENTS OF FITNESS These are the major components of physical fitness — (i) Cardiorespiratory Endurance – Cardiorespiratory system is the interrelated collective system of heart, lungs and blood vessels. Cardiorespiratory fitness or aerobic fitness depends upon heart's ability to pump oxygen-rich blood to the working muscles and utilization of oxygen by the working muscles. Cardiorespiratory endurance training should always find a proper place in your exercise programme and should be done 3-5 days in a week, depending on your specific goal. (ii) Muscular strength – It is the maximal ability of a muscle (or muscle group) to generate force. In simple words, it means the maximum weight you can lift during a single repetition. It is measured in RM (repetition maximum 3). 1 RM bench press or 1 RM squat is good way to test your upper and lower body strength respectively. (iii) Muscular Endurance – Muscular endurance is the ability of a muscle (or muscle group) to generate force repeatedly for a longer time. Although muscular strength and muscular endurance are related, they are not the same. An example of muscular strength is a person lifting heavy barbell during one maximal effort. In contrast, muscular endurance is illustrated by a person performing maximum number of repetitions of Chin ups, abdominal curl ups, push ups etc. (iv) Agility – Agility is one's ability for quick start, quick stop, and quick change of direction. Agility is very important in games. A more agile boxer would save himself more from his opponent's punches and land more punches on his opponent. (v)

Speed – Speed is one's ability to 'explode' (move fast) from one point to another point within shortest time. This is an all out effort. (vi) Flexibility – Flexibility can be defined as the ability to move joints through their full range of motion (ROM). Lack of flexibility training may shorten tendons and make them tight. Low flexibility is one of the major causes of injury. It is interesting to see some body builders moving like 'robots' with their rigid limbs. This is because of their lack of sufficient flexibility training. (vii) Body composition – Having right proportion of fat and lean body mass is an important component of fitness4 . (Total body mass includes fat and lean body mass. Lean body mass includes everything other than fat, viz., bones, water, protein, minerals). V. FITT FACTORS The acronym FITT stands for Frequency, Intensity, Time and Type (of exercise). It is important to keep these factors in mind while designing your exercise programme. Frequency It pays well to exercise the same muscle / muscle group frequently, 3- 5 days a week, and to have two days off for recovery. While less than required frequency will yield very marginal benefits, too much of frequency may result in overtraining.Intensity Intensity refers to the degree of effort. Intensity in cardiorespiratory endurance is measured by heart rate. Low intensity endurance training means training at low heart rate. As the intensity of training goes up, heart rate also goes up. Similarly, intensity in strength training refers to the load or resistance. Low intensity strength training means training with low resistance or low weights. Intensity in this case is measured by the maximum number of repetitions, popularly referred as RM (repetition maximum). Thus 5 RM would mean that one can do maximum 5 repetitions with a particular weight. Higher the intensity, lower would be the R M. (Naturally !) Selection and progression in intensity will depend upon your exercise goal. For example, if your goal is to increase your muscular endurance, select a weight that allows you a 12+ R M. However, exercising at this intensity will have little effect on your muscle strength. To gain muscle strength you will have to increase the intensity that allows you 3-5 RM. Similarly, for cardiorespiratory endurance, major part of your training should consist of building aerobic base at low intensity. But to reduce your race time you will have to increase the training intensity e.g., by including interval runs. (See section on Running). Also, follow the principle of progression while increasing your training intensity and avoid 'too much too soon' approach. Time (duration) This is one of the most frequently asked questions – what should be the minimum or maximum duration of exercise for maximum gains? Well, the answer is

– it all depends upon your training goal, and availability of time. On one hand, there are professionals who train 5-6 hours daily; on the other hand, there are executives who hardly find more than 20-30 minutes to spare for physical training. If your goal is just to keep fit, and you have 17 only 20-30 minutes, a circuit training consisting of one or two sets of muscle strength / endurance training of all major muscles / muscle groups may be the answer5 . But if you really want to improve your cardiorespiratory endurance or muscle strength or flexibility, you need to invest a little more time in training. For good cardiorespiratory endurance, one requires to do at least 20- 30 minutes of continuous training. This excludes time for warm-up, cooldown and stretching. For muscle strength one needs to perform at least 3- 5 sets of the same exercise. Total exercise time depends upon the number of repetitions, sets and recovery time taken between two sets. Similarly, each flexibility exercise also may require minimum 15-30 seconds, depending upon the type of stretch. If you have to cut short your time on exercise, do so on the total number of repetitions /sets, but never compromise on the recovery time. Rushing through the 'rituals' of all exercises hurriedly without allowing recovery may result into undue fatigue and injury. Type There are different types of exercises e.g., walking, running, stair climbing, bicycling, rowing, swimming, etc., for cardiorespiratory endurance; free weights, resistance machines, free hand etc., for muscular strength / endurance; stretches, Yogasanas for flexibility. The selection of a particular type or a combination of more than one type depends upon your exercise goal. For example, if your goal is to excel in running, focus on running; swimming is not going to help you much. Likewise, for a discuss thrower, cardiorespiratory endurance exercises may not be of much help; he has to focus more on strength training and flexibility training. Availability of resources may be sometimes a crucial factor in selection of a particular type/types of exercise.

VI. WARM-UP AND COOL-DOWN A. Warm-up – Systematic and sufficient warm-up is a must before starting any vigorous exercise session. Warm-up consists of a set of continuous exercises, which are done with a gradual build-up of speed to elevate body's core temperature till the point of perspiration. Beginning of perspiration is a good indicator that we are sufficiently warmed-up. During warming-up the temperature of muscles increases. A warmed-up muscle contracts and relaxes more quickly. Secondly, warming-up also helps more blood flow to the muscles. More blood flow means supply of more oxygen to muscles and hence more energy is available for exercise. Thirdly, our ligaments, tendons lose their stiffness and become more stretchable. Fourthly, our joints become more flexible. All these prevent possible injury caused by sudden load of high intensity exercise caused by high speed or heavy weight. No warm-up session is complete without stretching. Some people start warm-up session with stretching. This is not a proper way to start. In absence of sufficient elevation of our core temperature, our muscles, ligaments, tendons would remain stiff. If we stretch them in this condition, we would make them more susceptible to injury. Therefore, proper sequence of warm-up procedure would be to start with some easy slow body movements, gradually increasing the speed till the point of perspiration and then following it by stretching. Types of warm-up (i) Passive warm-up – In passive warm-up temperature of muscles is increased by outside efforts, e.g., by giving vigorous massage or hot baths. This is not always practical. (ii) General warm-up – It involves movement of maximum number of muscles for overall warm-up. Slow jog followed by 20-30 metre 19 sprints, cycling, skipping, climbing hill or stairs, etc. are a few activities for general warm-up. (iii) Specific warm-up – Before loading a specific muscle with high intensity exercise, it is advisable to warm-up that specific muscle. For example, slow jog will be good before starring a run. Light repetitions of bench press or a few push-ups will be helpful to lift a heavy weight afterwards. Warm-up process may take slightly more time in a cold weather. Better conditioned sportspersons are also likely to take more time. Nevertheless, warm-up is too important to be overlooked. B. Cool-down – Cool-down is reverse process of warm-up. While warm-up may be compared to pre-take-off run of an aeroplane, cool-down is like its taxiing after the landing. The same set of exercises used for warmup can be used for cool-down also. It involves gradual decrease in the intensity of exercise before stopping completely. Cool-down allows increased heart rate and blood pressure to gradually come down to normal level. Cool-down process should be concluded with stretching. In fact, stretching is more important during cool-down than during warm-up. It helps to reduce blood pooling in exercised muscles and removes lactic acid build-up (which is the immediate cause of tiredness and discomfort). In absence of proper cool-down, we may feel discomforts like headache, nausea, cramps, at the end of intense exercise and stiffness of muscles, tendons subsequently. VII. INJURY MANAGEMENT Causes – 99% of our injuries during exercise are result of our own carelessness and violation of the basic principles of exercise. Injury may occur due to incorrect form and or technique, 'too much too soon' approach, low level of experience, medical history, low fitness level combined with overtraining, inadequate recovery time, lack of proper 20 nutrition, insufficient or no warm-up/cool-down, poor concentration, adverse environment, failure to understand warning signs of body. Injury may also occur due to malfunctioning of exercise equipment, cluttered gym, etc. Prevention – Injury is largely preventable if we follow these guidelines – (i) Purchase good quality equipment, training apparels including shoes. (ii) Never ignore warm-up and cool-down. (iii) Use proper form and technique. (iv) Follow the basic principles of exercise. (v) Get assistance of a spotter in case of lifting heavy weights. (vi) Focus your mind on the exercise, especially during high-intensity exercise. Focus of mind not only protects you against injury, it also enhances your performance. (vii) Take sufficient precautions against extreme environment (heat, cold). (viii) Take proper nutrition. For example, lack of required protein may impair muscle growth and its repair. (ix) Slight discomfort or agony during exercise is OK and desirable. However, any kind of joint or muscular pain should be treated as a signal to stop or slow down. (x) When you resume exercise after a long gap, start from a lower degree of intensity / volume and gradually reach the standard you had achieved when you had left training. (xi) Avoid jerky movements in weight training. All movements should be at a controlled, slow, smooth pace. (xii) Stop exercise at once on warning signs of dizziness, acute fatigue, mental confusion. (xiii) Flexibility prevents injury. Do include flexibility in your exercise session. (xiv) In case of long-duration (more than 30-40 minutes) exercise, hydrate yourself well at frequent intervals. 21 (xv) In case of an injury, don't deny your injury. Discontinue exercise and seek proper medical help to avoid further worsening of injury. Management – In case of injury apply the principle of RICE (Rest, Ice, Compression, Elevation). Rest – Give rest to the injured part. Ice – Apply ice to the injured area. Cooling by ice decreases swelling of the affected part. Ice can be applied for 10-15 minutes at interval of 30-40 minutes. Compression – Compress the affected area with a firm but not too tight elastic bandage. Elevation – During first 24-72 hrs elevation of the affected part helps in checking swelling by reducing the blood flow. Remember, RICE is a first aid only. Don't hesitate to consult a doctor in case your injury prolongs. Injury of any part of the body does not necessarily mean complete abandon of exercise. Unless medically advised otherwise, one can exercise one's unaffected body parts. For example, if your shoulders are injured, there is no reason why you cannot exercise your legs, abdominal muscles, forearms. Overtraining – Overtraining is generally caused by our 'too much too soon' approach to exercise. Inappropriately high levels of intensity or volume of exercise, or both combined together, and insufficient recovery time lead to overtraining. Neglect of proper nutrition is another significant factor that contributes to this phenomenon. One important sign of overtraining is that despite regular training, gains are stopped at a point and even worse, performance starts to decline. Other psychosomatic symptoms of overtraining are – ? Chronic muscle soreness/ joint pain, unduly nagging fatigue ? Stress-induced injury like tiny fractures ? Lack of enthusiasm for work out ? Lack of concentration 22 ? Irritability ? Sleep disorders ? Decrease in lean body mass (decrease in muscle mass) ? Decrease appetite ? Lowered immunity level ? Frequent cold-like symptoms ? Altered blood pressure ? Altered resting heart rate (RHR) An increase of more than 5 beats per minute above your normal (RHR) 6 may be an indication that you have done too much exercise on the previous day. So, next day either do little training or simply take rest. VIII. ENVIRONMENTAL CONSIDERATIONS Heat It is important to maintain our body's normal range of core temperature (36.1° - 37.8° C). Any excessive variation on either side of this range may affect our training performance and if not regulated, it may lead to injury also. During excessive heat (which may be caused by outside temperature or by high intensity of the exercise itself) our body starts sweating for cooling. However, sweating as a cooling mechanism of body has certain limitations. For example, during long bouts of exercise, as body's water contents deplete, the rate of sweating also declines and it becomes less effective as a cooling mechanism. Similarly, cooling effect of sweating also depends upon the relative humidity of air. Higher the air humidity, less will be the sweat evaporation (as air is saturated) and consequent cooling of body will be less. (Recall the experience with desert coolers during humid months). Thus, it is quite possible to feel more uncomfortable to run at 35° C on a humid day than to run at 40° C on a hot but dry day. Exercising in excessive heat may cause heat cramps (muscle cramps in arms, legs or abdomen), dehydration (symptoms like fatigue, dizziness, rapid pulse rate, weakness), heat exhaustion (weakness, excessive sweating, low blood pressure, dizziness) or heat stroke (high body temperature, rapid pulse, stoppage of sweating, mental confusion, disorientation, hallucinations). Children and elderly persons are particularly more susceptible to heat induced injuries as their body has less sweating capacity. Heat induced injuries, if not treated on time, may be fatal. Therefore, once the symptoms appear, exercise should be immediately stopped and medical help should be taken. Heat-related injuries may be prevented by (i) drinking water before and during exercising in the sun; (ii) drinking appropriate sports drinks to maintain electrolyte balance in the body; (iii) avoiding exposure to excessive heat and doing exercise during cooler part of the day; (iv) wearing light, porous clothes that promote fast sweat evaporation; (v) reducing the intensity and volume of exercise. On humid days, it is advisable to exercise at lower intensity. Take time to acclimatize to hot days. Cold Mildly cold winter mornings are probably the most enjoyable part of the year to train. However, the problem starts in extreme cold when the body heat loss is greater than body heat production. This condition may occur due to either extreme cold or insufficient clothing or very low intensity of exercise. Exposure to severe cold may lead to hypothermia, frostbite or dehydration. Wind worsens the situation during cold. Here again, children and elderly are more susceptible to risks of cold related injury as their body cannot produce metabolic heat that effectively. 24 Exercising during cold is a good idea to retain one's normal range of core body temperature. However, once exercise is stopped, exposure to sweat-soaked clothing may lead to hypothermia. Therefore, it is advisable to (i) do low intensity exercise to avoid excessive sweating; (ii) wear porous clothes to allow maximum sweat evaporation; (iii) change into a set of dry clothes immediately after the exercise. Do not forget to change socks and undergarments. Wearing track suit throughout the exercise session is not of much use. Once you are sufficiently warmed up, remove your track suit and exercise in normal one-layer apparel to allow sweat evaporation. Once you stop exercising, again wear the track suit to keep body warm. Cold related injuries can be prevented by wearing suitable multiple layers of clothing. Multiple layers of thin clothing are more effective in retaining heat than single thick-layered clothing. A good amount of heat loss occurs through open head, neck and hands. Therefore, these exposed body parts should be properly covered. In extreme cold, wearing an additional pair of socks and undergarments will be helpful. Our subcutaneous fat is an excellent insulator against cold. This makes skinny models (who have very low fat mass) more vulnerable to cold related injuries in comparison with others who have normal % body fat. Another interesting thing about cold is that for its maintenance our body utilizes more carbohydrate and fat than in summer. So, winter is a good time to work out hard, eat heartily and still be in shape! High Altitude At high altitudes our performance decreases mainly due to presence of less oxygen. Before starting serious training, therefore one should take 3-4 weeks time to acclimatize by progressively increasing the intensity and volume of exercise. If not sufficiently acclimatized, one may get headache, nausea, loss of appetite, sleep disorders, etc. 25 Pollution When pollution level is very high outside, it is better to exercise indoors. Pollution is more harmful if you are doing a serious endurance training as it involves breathing through mouth. As you know, our mouth, unlike our nostrils, does not have any natural filter against pollutants. Therefore, select a time and place for exercise where pollution level is relatively low. It is relevant to mention here that quality of indoor air – whether inside your house, office or gym – is an important issue. Moisture, pets, dust mites, materials used in household furnishings, e.g., mattresses, curtains, carpets, etc. are some of the major sources of poor quality indoor air. These may cause minor allergies and may aggravate respiratory problems. By providing proper ventilation, allowing sunshine to enter into the room, regular cleaning of furnishings, replacing carpets with hard surface tiles (which are easy to clean), regular cleaning of air conditioners, coolers etc. we can reduce the pollution level indoors. IX. WOMEN AND EXERCISE As men are generally bigger than women in size, their greater strength compared to women's is mainly due to their larger size and hence greater muscle mass. There is no difference in muscle response of men and women and both can benefit in the same manner from a similar exercise programme. Generally, women are more flexible than men. Women have 25% smaller heart and 25-30% less lung capacity than that of men. Smaller heart means that it would have to work more to pump the same amount of blood. This combined with less lung capacity implies that women will fatigue faster than men. But this holds good only when we compare a woman with equally trained man. This should not, however, give men a false sense of superiority over women. A well-trained woman can beat an untrained/under-trained man in all aspects of physical fitness. 26 Women can exercise during menstruation. Pregnant women also can exercise, though with medical advice. Vigorous activity does not have any adverse effect on women's reproductive organs or menstruation. There should be no undue concern about post-partum (after delivery of a child) fitness of women unless there have been other medical complications associated with it. There are many top 'mother' athletes in all sports and games. As regards apparels, proper sports bras are advised for women to prevent any damage to their breasts tissue during exercise causing prolonged jarring of breasts (e.g., in long distance running). Similarly, men are also advised to wear properly fitted underwears/supporters during such exercises. Some women, especially long distance runners, may experience menstrual irregularities. Possible explanation for this is temporary sharp decline in estrogen production which is linked with fall in body fat below a certain level. Low-calorie intake and other nutritional deficiencies may be some of other factors causing menstrual irregularities. However, it is a temporary phenomenon and with restoration of normal fat percentage, normalcy is restored. Many women fear that strength training would make them too muscular and give them a 'manly' look. This fear is unfounded as the muscle size of a woman cannot increase much beyond a point. Women (as well as men) who are obsessed with weight control, often rely more on cardio-vascular exercise combined with low calorie diet. They ignore strength training and flexibility training. Such practice is against the basic principles of exercise. Avoiding strength training will deprive women of all its related benefits, viz., strengthening of muscle, bone, ligaments, tendons, etc. Bigger muscles help in weight control as they increase RMR of the body. Higher RMR means more caloric expenditure. Low calories intake decreases RMR and thus decrease the rate of weight loss. These 27 things have been further explained in the chapter on Weight Management. There is another misconception that strength training would turn fat into muscle. It is impossible as these two are quite different. Strength training increases size of muscles fibres, not of fat cells. X. CHILDREN AND EXERCISE Moderate strength exercise, e.g., push ups, chin ups, squatting does not affect children adversely. It does not blunt their growth. It rather helps them to perform better in their school sports. However, intensive strength training involving heavy weights is not recommended for children on two grounds– (i)they may overtrain themselves without realizing its adverse implications and (ii) they may not follow the correct form and technique making themselves more vulnerable to injuries or deformities caused by repetitive use of wrong technique over a period of time. As far as endurance training is concerned, studies suggest that children should not train intensively before age 18. Hard training before this age may result into their early burn outs. Intensive endurance training combined with low calorie diet may further cause damage to them. Therefore, it is advised, once they are mature, they can train hard. Speed training is more advisable for children. They should be encouraged to participate in a variety of games and sports for overall fitness and normal growth. XI. ELDERLY AND EXERCISE Exercise is beneficial at any age. It is never too late to start exercise. And there is no reason to stop it at any age. Look at Baba Fauja Singh (born 1911), who set up a marathon world record of 5 hours 40 minutes in 2003 in the 90 plus age category. He re-discovered his passion for running at 81. Manohar Aich (born 1912), nicknamed 'Pocket Hercules', the first 28 Mr. Universe (1952) from India, was another example of what elderly can do. WHO (World Health Organization) recommends that older adults should engage in at least 30 minutes of moderate intensity physical activity 5 days per week. In fact, there are no specific advices to elderly than for anyone else. Whether adult or elderly, the only point to remember is – follow the basic principles of exercise. Elderly should have a thorough physical examination before starting an intensive strength or endurance training. Older adults must realize that with age their age-predicted maximal heart rate (APMHR or MHR)7 declines. APMHR = 220 – age. Therefore, know your training heart rate (THR)8 (see section on Endurance Training) and exercise within the limit. The body of an elderly takes more time to adapt to increased intensity and volume of exercise. It implies that your progression may be slower and recovery period may be longer. Degree of (physical) balance declines in old age. Some of the bathroom falls may be avoided by ensuring good balance exercises. A few practical exercises can be done in day-to-day life to improve balance, e.g., taking off shoes while standing, standing on one leg and lifting the other upto knee level, (or, doing the same exercise with eyes closed) etc. Aerobic exercise, e.g., brisk walk, jogging, cycling, swimming, etc., is an effective tool for weight management because it increases our total daily caloric expenditure. However, one must include some sort of strength training in his exercise programme because only strength training can slow down age-related decline in muscle mass, bone mass and overall strength.

XII. EXERCISE APPARELS Clothing Clothing should be comfortable and should not restrict any movement of body during exercise. A good quality non-cotton T-shirt or sleeveless undershirt and gym shorts are best in warm weather. Light, porous clothing such as 'fish net' vests allow sweat to come on their outer surface and evaporate quickly, thus promoting faster heat loss from our body. (Such T-shirts and shorts are available in local markets and also in almost all brands, e.g., 'Climalite' (Adidas), 'Dri fit' (Nike) etc.). On the other hand, cotton T-shirts become soggy (heavy with water) after absorbing sweat and make a layer that prevents adequate heat loss from our body. The recommendation for polyester vests/T-shirts might sound strange, as we have always been advised to prefer cotton clothes. Yes, cotton clothes are preferable for their sweat-absorbing quality when we have to sit in the office where we do not sweat much, but polyester/nylon clothes are preferable during exercise for their faster heat loss facilitation quality. Light-material sleeveless vests/shorts are easy to maintain, as they hardly require any ironing. They can be daily washed after one use (unlike track lowers, which are generally washed after 2-3 or even more usage). We should also not forget about the decency of our wears. During winter, clothing should be both insulating and ventilating. It is better to wear more than one layer of clothing than to wear single thick clothing. Upto 40% of heat loss may take place through head, neck and hands when uncovered. Therefore, in case of extreme cold, head, neck and hands should be well covered. Shoes Choice of appropriate shoes can prevent one from many runninginduced injuries. There are hundreds of varieties of shoes available in the 30 market in different price categories. While money is a factor, one should not save money on shoes only to later spend more (money as well as peace of mind) on treatment of injury! Therefore, choice is very clear – invest reasonable amount of money on purchase of good shoes, enjoy an injuryfree running or buy a cheap pair of shoes, injure yourself and then go on spending more money on treatment of your injury! Generally, while buying shoes, keep the following points in mind – (i) Try shoes in the afternoon. The size of shoes should be slightly larger than your normal use conventional shoes. (Buy 9½ -10-No. running shoes, if you generally wear 9-No. shoes). This is because your foot swells during the day and during running. (ii) When trying on shoes, wear socks in which you will run. Also, try on both shoes, as our feet slightly differ in size and shape. (iii) Shoes must have proper arch support and heel-cushioning. (iv) Feel the seams inside for ensuring that they are smooth. (v) Shoes are not to be used for running after approx. 800-1000 kms of running. (vi) The width of the toe box should be sufficient to allow easy toe movement inside (vii) Shoes with extensive toe box netting material allow faster heat loss through evaporation of sweat. (viii) Never ignore the quality of socks. Cushioned socks function as additional shock absorbers during running. XIII.EXERCISE PROGRAMME DESIGN For optimal results, any fitness training programme design must take care of (a) basic principles of exercise, (b) FITT factors and (c) major 31 components of fitness. This can be better understood by the table given below – If you have a 6-day exercise regimen; Monday, Wednesday and Friday may be devoted to cardiovascular fitness and Tuesday, Thursday and Saturday for muscle strength / endurance. Sunday can be the rest day. In case of a 5-day regimen, in the first week Monday, Wednesday and Friday may be kept for cardiovascular fitness and Tuesday and Thursday for muscle strength /endurance. Saturday and Sunday may be the rest days. In the next week, the training days are flip-flopped, i.e., muscle strength/endurance can be done on Monday, Wednesday and Friday and cardiovascular on Tuesday, Thursday and so on. Stretching should be done in every training session, during warm-up, during exercise (between two sets) and during cool-down. Earmarking number of days for strength or endurance training depends on your training goal. If you are primarily focusing on strength, you may like to devote four days to strength training and two days to endurance training, and vice versa. 9. HRR is heart rate reserve is the difference between one's MHR and RHR. (HRR= MHR-RHR) 10. RM – Repetition Maximum. 11, 12. See 'Types of stretching' in the chapter Flexibility Training. FITT Components of fitness Cardiorespiratory Endurance Muscular Strength Muscular Endurance Flexibility Frequency 3-5 times/ week 3 times/ week 3-5 times/ week Everyday Intensity 60-90% HRR9 3-6 RM10 12-15 RM Till the point of slight discomfort but NOT PAIN Time 20-30 minutes or more The time required to do 3-6 repetitions of each exercise The time required to do 12-15 repetitions of each exercise 20-30 seconds each stretch Type Running Swimming Bicycling Jumping Rope Walking/Hiking Stair Climbing Free Weights Resistance Machines Partner-Resisted Exercises Body-Weight Exercises (Pushups/Situps/Pullups/Dips, etc.) Active11 Passive12 32 Here are some other important tips for an effective exercise programme design – ? Firstly, decide about your specific goal. ? Keep in your mind total availability of time. ? Never skip warm-up / cool-down for lack of time. If you do not have enough time, better you reduce the number of sets rather than reducing warm-up session. ? If you resume your exercise after a long lay off (due to illness, job engagement etc.,) start from a lower intensity/volume so as to condition yourself before you reach your pre-lay off level. This will save you from injury. ? Monitor your progress. If you have reached your training plateau or your performance is declining, then redesign the exercise programme. ? Keep scope for occasional games and sports for variety and freshness. ? Include Yogic breathing, i.e., Pranayam in your exercise routine.

CHAPTER FOUR

STRENGTH TRAINING

Strength is the ability to produce a force. Strength training consists of resistance exercises1 , which increase one's muscle strength, muscle size, speed and power. I. BENEFITS OF STRENGTH TRAINING These are some major benefits of strength training – (i) It benefits individuals of all age. (ii) It increases muscle strength, muscle endurance and muscle power. (iii) Increased muscle mass causes increased resting metabolic rate (RMR) and consequent increased total daily energy expenditure. This helps in weight management. (iv) It slows down the process of sarcopenia (loss of muscle mass in older adults) by increasing muscle mass. (v) It strengthens our bones by loading them and thereby increasing bone density. The risk of bone fracture by falling in old age is thus reduced. (vi) It helps us carry out our day-to-day work easily. (vii) It improves stability, balance, posture and boosts up our selfconfidence.STRENGTH TRAINING EXERCISE TECHNIQUES Remember the following basics of strength training techniques – (i) Assume correct body form and maintain it throughout the exercise. (ii) Know about the muscles to be targeted and focus on them while exercising. (iii) Proper breathing is very important during exercise. Here, the simple rule is this – Breathe out during the hardest part of the exercise and breathe in during the easier part of the exercise. For example, during bench press, breathe out while lifting the weight and breathe in while lowering the weight. But at no point, you should forcibly hold your breath. Holding breath can induce excessive increase in blood pressure. Dizziness, sudden loss of strength would be warning signs. In such a situation, immediately stop exercise. (iv) Use weightlifting belts in case of lifting maximal or near-maximal weight while doing structural exercises. Structural exercises are those exercises which load your trunk and place stress on the lower back (e.g., squat, standing shoulder press, dead lift, etc.). However, use of weightlifting belt for even lighter weights may cause under-exercise and related under-strengthening of muscles of lower back and abdomen. Such weaker torso-muscles may get injured, in case a heavier weight is lifted without weightlifting belts. III. STRENGTH TRAINING PROGRAMME DESIGN A strength training programme should be guided primarily by one's training goal. Broadly, training goals may fall into one of these categories – (i) muscular strength (ii) muscular endurance (iii) hypertrophy (increased muscle size). A common man or woman may be happy with just overall fitness. Athletes and sportspersons will do it for improving their sports 35 performance. Professionals like members of police or army may find it useful to achieve prescribed physical fitness standards set for them. Like any other exercise programme, strength training also should take into account the following principles of exercise/ FITT factors – A. Specificity – Identify your training goals. Identify the muscles that come into play in your specific game, sports or job. Select specific exercises that target those relevant muscle groups. Beginners should select exercises to workout their all important large and small muscles for overall conditioning, viz., chest, shoulders, upper back, lower back, thighs, calves, abdomen, biceps and triceps. Afterwards, they can select specific exercises as per their goal. B. Frequency – When we say that strength training should be done 3-5 times a week, we mean that the strength training of the same muscle group has to be done 3-5 times a week. There should be a recovery gap of 48-72 hours (not less than one day and more than two days) between two sessions. A beginner can have two sessions in a week (e.g., Monday and Thursday) or three sessions (e.g., Monday, Wednesday and Friday). Advanced trainees can have workouts on three days. A split routine allows them four or more sessions also. However, it is important to avoid workout of the same muscle groups on two days in a row. Workouts may be planned thus – Upper body on Monday and Thursday; lower body on Tuesday and Friday. There may be several other combinations depending upon your time constraints. C. Progression – Once you overload your system, your muscles would adapt to it by increasing their strength. If you continue your training with the same load, (i.e., same number of repetitions /sets with same weight), you will not gain further. Therefore, go on increasing your training load to reach your full training potential. 36 How do you know that it is time to increase the load? 2-for-2-rule may help you in this regard. According to this rule, if you can complete 02 more repetitions than the repetition goal in the final set of an exercise for 02 consecutive training sessions, the load in all sets of that exercise should be increased in the next training session. For example, if your repetition goal is 10 in an exercise and you can complete 2 more repetitions (i.e., 12 repetitions) in the final set in two consecutive training sessions, it is time to increase load during the next training session. The next question comes – how much weight should you increase? The answer is, increase the weight with which you can perform minimum number of required repetitions of your target range. For example, if your target range of repetitions is 8-10 per set, you should be able to perform minimum 8 repetitions with the increased weight. D. Overload – Overloading in strength training can be done by (i) increasing weight/resistance, (ii) increasing total number repetitions/sets, (iii) reducing recovery time between two sets, (iv) reducing repetition velocity by slowing down muscle movement. (For example, while doing bench press, take 8 seconds (instead of usual 4 seconds) to lower down the weight.) It is important to perform all repetitions while strictly maintaining correct form and technique. Secondly, required number of repetitions should be done till total muscle failure. Total muscle failure occurs when one cannot do another correct repetition anymore. Never distort your body and compromise with the correct form just to perform one or two additional repetitions. You will gain nothing but injury by doing so. The number of repetitions and sets depends upon your primary training goal. Beginners may benefit even with one set (during initial 3-4 weeks). However, you will have to perform 2-6 sets to reach your full 37 potential. Select a weight that allows you to do prescribed range of repetitions. The following guidelines will be useful in this regard – It is important to perform the same number of repetitions in each set. It may happen that the fatigue caused by the earlier set may not allow you to perform the same number of repetitions in the subsequent set. Then you have two options to reach your repetitions goal – (i) take assistance of your partner (spotter), or, (ii) drop some load and perform the target number of repetitions. E. Recovery – Duration of recovery period between two sets is an important factor in strength training. For endurance, sets (with light weight) are performed in quick succession allowing little rest between two sets. For strength, sets (with heavy weight) are performed allowing full rest between two sets. General guidelines in this regard are given in the following table – With experience you will learn about the optimal rest period for you. Full rest means when your rate of breathing becomes normal. F. Variation – Performance of the same set of exercises for a long time may result into overtraining or undertraining of particular muscle groups and boredom of the trainee – all resulting into a decline in performance. The remedy is to introduce variation in exercises. For example, different Training Goal Repetitions Sets Muscular endurance ≥ 12 2-3 Hypertrophy (increased muscle size as in body building) 6-12 3-6 Muscular strength ≤ 6 2-6 Training Goal Rest Period Length Muscular endurance ≤ 30 seconds Hypertrophy (body building) 30-90 seconds Muscular strength 2-5 minutes 38 training days may be marked as heavy, medium, light training day when the load would be heavy, medium and light respectively, though number of repetitions may be the same. G. Balance – While principle of specificity in strength training is important, equally important is the element of balance. Never ignore any muscle group completely, even though you may like to focus on specific muscle group, train the whole body. There should be a balance between upper body and lower body. To ensure a balanced workout, do at least one set of exercise for each of the major muscle group. Important – A strong lower back adds considerably to our overall strength and protects us against lower back injuries, yet sometimes it is the most neglected area. Never ignore your lower back. In our day to day life, lower back injuries are one of the most common injuries. They occur due to (a) weak lower back and abdominal muscles and (b) wrong form and technique of lifting weight. I will go to the extent to recommend that, if you have only 5-10 minutes to spare for exercise, exercise your lower back and abdominal muscles only. Strong lower back and abdominal muscles are great support for the spine. In absence of strong supporting muscles the spine will have to bear the maximum load by itself and therefore would be susceptible to injury. IV. SEQUENCE OF EXERCISE Follow these guidelines – (i) The most important point is that exercises should be ordered in such a manner that fatigue caused by the previous exercise either (a) does not affect or (b) affects your strength for subsequent exercise the least. One way to ensure this is to alternate e.g., upper body exercise followed by lower body exercise, again upper body exercise, and so on. This sequence gives the exercised muscle enough time to recover 39 between two sets. The sample circuit training given in Appendix-I is based on this principle. (ii) Start with core exercises2 and then proceed to assistance exercises3 . In other words, larger muscle groups should be addressed first followed by smaller muscles. V. SAFETY FACTORS Strength training is thoroughly enjoyable and safe. Injuries happen mostly because of neglect of certain basic safety rules. Make sure you follow these safety rules – (i) Warm up well before starting the training. (ii) Focus you mind especially while lifting heavy weights. (iii) Always use proper form and technique. (iv) Avoid 'too much too soon' approach. (v) Have a spotter (partner) especially during lifting of heavy free weights. (vi) Never hold your breath while lifting weights. (vii) Obey the discipline of gym. Don't leave weights, bars, etc. unattended on floor.

FREE HAND EXERCISES Here is a list of free hand exercises with full description of their technique, variations, etc. The same set of exercises can be used for both muscular strength training as well as muscular endurance training. You can use them for strength training in these ways – (i) Slow down the movement, e.g., take 6-8 seconds to lower down instead of usual 2 seconds while performing push-us, squats, chinups, etc. (ii) Pause at the peak of each repetition for 2 seconds. (iii) Ask your partner to increase the load by applying pressure on you throughout the movement. The load should be such as to allow you maximum 3-6 repetitions in a set. Follow the overload principle mentioned under Strength Training Programme Design. (iv) Adopt more difficult variations. (v) Take sufficient recovery time in between. Familiarity with major muscles of human body will help you to be more systematic and focused.

Push-ups Areas worked – Pectorals, deltoids, upper back, triceps and abdominals. Technique ? Assume the position as in . Feet 10-12 inches apart. Hands 4- 5 inches wider than shoulder width. Body straight. Stomach pulled in. ? Lower your body slowly till your chest touches the ground (Peak) . ? Push your body up to the original position . (This is 01 repetition). ? Do required number of repetitions. ? Keep your body straight throughout the movement. Don'ts ? Don't arch your lower back. This may unduly stress your lower back. ? Don't let your body 'fall'. Lower your body in a slow, controlled way. ? Don't hold your breath at any point of time.

Hints and Tips ? Use bricks to rest your hands for greater range of movement of your muscles. ? Place your feet on a chair or bed to work out your upper chest . Gradually you can increase the elevation and finally do push ups with legs supported against a wall. Take care not to get dizzy. ? Increase the width of hands for wider push-ups . ? Perform push-ups with your hands closed together or 2-3 inches apart. This is an excellent exercise for triceps. ? Tell your partner to apply pressure on your upper back to increase load throughout the movement.

Variation (a) Power push ups are more difficult variation of push ups. Technique ? Rest your hands on a medicine ball . (Place the ball in a shallow pit for stability). ? Move your hands off the ball and quickly place them on ground at shoulder width, simultaneously lowering down the body till your chest almost touches the ball . ? Push your body back to the original position . (This is 01 repetition). ? Do required number of repetitions. ? Keep your body straight throughout the movement. ? Alternatively, acquire the standard push-ups position as in . Push your body up, clap in the air and again come back to the original position . ? Keep your body straight throughout the movement.

SQUATS

Shallow dive push-ups are another variation of push-ups, which are very popular among traditional wrestlers. I have found that this variation of push-ups addresses more muscle groups of upper body than the standard push-ups. Technique ? Acquire the position . ? Lower down your body, move forward and up as if you are diving into and emerging from water . ? Come back to the original position.

Take care not to make any jerky movement. There should be no stress on lower back at all

If you ever watch toddlers move, you'll notice that they execute picture-perfect squats time and again. But when you're well into adulthood, how to do squats becomes a little more of a loaded question: Are your feet in the right position? Are you getting down far enough? Should you add weight?

While there's a lot to unpack with how to do a proper squat, the benefits of learning how to squat correctly are immense—squat variations not only help you get stronger during your workouts, but they also represent a movement pattern that you use during everyday life.

"In life, we squat all the time, from playing with our children to going to the bathroom to sitting on a chair, " Noam Tamir, C.S.C.S., founder and CEO of TS Fitness in New York City, tells SELF. "It's very much a functional movement."

When you learn how to do squats correctly, you can really make the most out of the move—and your workout. Here's what you need to know.

What muscles do squats work, and what are the benefits of squats?

The squat is considered a compound movement, meaning it works multiple muscle groups across multiple joints. The primary muscles involved in the movement are your quadriceps (the muscles in the front of your thighs) and your glutes (your butt muscles), Tamir says. On the eccentric part of the move, or the lowering portion of the squat, the muscles in your hamstrings and your hip flexors fire too. Squats also work the muscles around the knee, which helps build strength and prevent injury, he says.

Throughout the move, your core muscles fire in order to keep you steady.

"Your abdominals are stabilizers," he says. "So they assist in weight-bearing movements." Strong core muscles are important because not only do they help you with your lifts, but they also reduce the risk of lower back pain.

If you do a weighted squat—whether using a dumbbell in a goblet squat, two dumbbells in a front squat, or a barbell in either a back or front squat—you're also working your upper body. That's because the move requires an isometric holding of weight, a static muscle contraction without any movement, Tamir says.

Weighted squats, like other forms of load-bearing physical activity, also benefit your bones: They help you build stronger bones, he says, which can help prevent osteopenia or osteoporosis as you get older.

Plus, since a proper squat requires mobility in your hips and ankles, you can also consider squatting a mobility exercise that can help you move better, Tamir says.

Everything you need to know about how to do squats

Before you start adding weight, you want to get the squat motion down with bodyweight squats first. Form is key, since performing squats properly can cut down the risk of injury during the move.

Here's what you need to know about doing squats correctly, and how you can avoid some common squatting mistakes.

1. Assume the squat stance.

Before you squat, you should get in proper squat position: Keep your feet about shoulder-width apart, Tamir says. There's no set rule for exact positioning of your feet—it'll vary depending upon anatomical differences—but a good guideline is for them to turn out anywhere between 5 and 30 degrees. So rather than pointing straight ahead, your feet will turn out slightly, but how much they do will depend on your particular comfort level and mobility.

2. Screw your feet into the floor.

Dialing your feet into the ground helps engage your muscles, improve alignment, and create stability with the ground, says Tamir. It'll also help keep your arches from collapsing, which can make your knees more likely to cave inward when you squat. (This is what's known as knee valgus.)

3. Keep your chest up.

Your upper body also matters for squats. "Keep your chest up, your chest proud," says Tamir. This will prevent your shoulders and upper back from rounding—a common mistake—which could overstress your spine, especially if you are squatting with weight on your back.

4. Initiate the movement.

When you're ready to squat, think about starting the movement by bending your knees and pushing your hips back, says Tamir. Engage your core for the descent, and keep it braced throughout the move.

"Make sure you're controlling the eccentric part of the movement," he says. Rather than rushing through the downward motion, take a couple of seconds to lower yourself. This will increase time under tension for your muscles, which will make them work harder. (Slowing down the eccentric is also a great strategy to make the move feel harder if you're working out at home and don't have access to the weights you're used to.)

Inhale while you lower, and as you squat down, your knees should track laterally above your first or second toe, Tamir says. Tracking too far in can also make your knees collapse inward, and tracking too far out can put extra stress on them. (Don't worry so much about the old rule that your knees should never extend forward farther than your toes, Tamir says. Knees extending farther than your toes can happen due to anatomical differences in your bone length. Trying to restrict that movement can actually make you lean forward more, which can stress your lower back, according to a study in the Journal of Strength and Conditioning Research.)

5. Pause when you reach parallel.

As for when you should stop the move? There's lots of discussion about how low you should squat, but the average exerciser should shoot to hit parallel depth with their squats, says Tamir. "That means the back of your thighs will be parallel to the floor," he says.

Some people have difficulty getting to parallel because of lack of mobility or injury—and if that's the case, it's better to end the squat at whatever depth is pain-free for you—but sometimes people default to quarter-squats because they're using too much weight, says Tamir. If that's the case, easing off the weight and performing the full range of motion for the move is optimal.

Once you reach the bottom of the squat, pause for a second so you are not using momentum to push yourself back up. (You can also increase the length of your pause to add difficulty to the move.)

6. When you stand, drive through your heels.

Make sure your feet stay planted throughout the duration of the squat, paying particular attention to driving through your heels on the way back up, says Tamir. This will fire up your posterior chain—the muscles in the back of your body, like your hamstrings and glutes.

Some people have a tendency to pick up their toes when they're focusing on driving through their heels, but you really want to make sure your entire foot stays firmly on the ground: "Your big toe is actually really important in glute activation," he says.

You should also exhale on your way back up, says Tamir. Making sure you breathe throughout the move—inhale on the way down, exhale on the way up—is vital. You definitely do not want to be holding your breath.

7. Finish strong.

At the top of the squat, try to tuck your pelvis into a neutral position. "Think of it like bringing your belt buckle to your chin," says Tamir. Just be careful that you are not hyperextending: A common mistake Tamir sees often is people pushing their hips too far forward, which can actually make you lean backward and stress your lower back.

What's the best way to progress with squats?

Before you start loading your squat, you should definitely get the bodyweight move down, says Tamir. (If you're having difficulty with the movement, you can hold on to a wall or, if you have access to it, a suspension trainer like a TRX, to get more comfortable with what it should feel like.)

In some cases, if you are still having difficulty with the move, holding a light weight—like a five-pound dumbbell or a 10-pound plate—in front of your body as a counterbalance can actually help you master the move, says Tamir. "It gives them more weight in front of their body, so they feel more comfortable pushing through the heels and pushing their butt back."

When you're ready to add more load, the goblet squat is a helpful next progression, since you're holding the weight in front of you, says Tamir. This helps you drop into the squat and keep weight on your heels. Keep your elbows and wrists stacked vertically—you don't want your elbows to flare out at your sides.

After a goblet squat, you can try a dumbbell front squat, where you hold two dumbbells at your shoulders. This squat variation tends to be a little easier than a kettlebell front squat, which requires some technique to align your wrists. Barbell back squats and front squats are more advanced, and it's super important you get your technique down before adding large amounts of load.

? You can hold a fixed object, e.g., window bar to maintain your balance during squats. ? Fold your hands overhead for greater difficulty. ? Occasionally, you can do squats while standing on your toes throughout. This exercise mainly strengthens quadriceps close to knees and partly calves. This also improves your overall balance.

Lunges Technique

Lunges are a popular strength training exercise among people wanting to strengthen, sculpt, and tone their bodies, while also improving overall fitness and enhancing athletic performance.

This resistance exercise is popular for its ability to strengthen your back, hips, and legs, while improving mobility and stability. Lunges are ideal for those wishing to get stronger and for current athletes, including runners and cyclists.

Continue reading to take a look at the benefits of lunges along with what muscles they target and a few variation options.

Benefits of performing lunges

1. Weight loss

Lunges work the large muscle groups in your lower body, which builds leans muscle and reduces body fat. This can increase your resting metabolism, which allows you to burn more calories and trim excess weight.

If you're looking to lose weight, push yourself to your outer limits by including lunges in a high-intensity circuit training routine using heavy weights.

2. Balance and stability

Lunges are a lower body unilateral exercise since you work on each side of your body independently. The single-leg movements activate your stabilizing muscles to develop balance, coordination, and stability.

Working one leg at a time causes your body to be less stable, which forces your spine and core to work harder to stay balanced.

3. Alignment and symmetry

Lunges are better than bilateral exercises for rehabilitation since they can correct imbalances and misalignments in your body to make it more symmetrical.

If you have one side that's less strong or flexible, spend a bit of extra time working on this side so you don't overcompensate or overuse the dominant side.

4. Stand taller

Lunges strengthen your back and core muscles without putting too much stress or strain on your spine. A strong, stable core reduces your chance of injury and improves your posture, making common movements easier.

Benefits by type of lunge

5. Stationary lunges

Stationary lunges target your glutes, quadriceps, and hamstrings. You'll put most of your weight on your front leg and use your back leg to balance, stabilize, and support your entire body.

You'll want to get the form down since stationary lunges are the foundation for all the lunge variations.

6. Side lunges

Lateral lunges develop balance, stability, and strength. They work your inner and outer thighs and may even help to reduce the appearance of cellulite.

Side lunges train your body to move side to side, which is a nice change from your body's normal forward or twisting movements. Plus, side lunges target your quadriceps, hips, and legs at a slightly different angle, thus working them a little differently.

Pay attention to the outsides of your legs and work on activating these muscles as you do these lunges.

7. Walking lunges

To do walking lunges, you'll need balance and coordination. The walking variation targets your core, hips, and glutes, and improves overall stability. They also increase your range of motion and help to improve your functional everyday movements.

To make walking lunges more difficult, add weights or a torso twist.

8. Reverse lunges

Reverse lunges activate your core, glutes, and hamstrings. They put less stress on your joints and give you a bit more stability in your front leg. This is ideal for people who have knee concerns, difficulty balancing, or less hip mobility.

Reverse lunges allow you to be more balanced as you move backward, changing up the direction from most of your movements and training your muscles to work differently.

9. Twist lunges

You can add a twist to stationary, walking, or reverse lunges to activate your core and glutes more deeply. Twisting lunges also require balance and stability as you twist your torso away from your lower body while maintaining the alignment of your knees.

You'll also activate the muscles in your ankles and feet.

10. Curtsy lunge

Curtsy lunges are great for strengthening and toning your derrière, which is excellent for your posture. Strong glutes also prevent and relieve back and knee pain, all of which help to improve your athletic performance and lower your risk of injury.

Curtsy lunges also sculpt and strengthen your hip adductors, quadriceps, and hamstrings as well as improve hip stabilization. Use a kettlebell or dumbbell to up the intensity of this variation.

11. Lunges and squats

Lunges and squats both work your lower body and are a valuable addition to your fitness regime. You may favor lunges if you have low back pain since they're less likely to strain your back. Consider focusing on squats if you feel more stable in this position.

Since this pair of exercises will work your body in similar ways, it's a matter of personal preference to see if either exercise feels better for your body or brings you the best results. Of course, adding both lunges and squats to your routine is beneficial.

Muscles worked

Lunges increase muscle mass to build up strength and tone your body, especially your core, butt, and legs. Improving your appearance isn't the main benefit of shaping up your body, as you'll also improve your posture and range of motion.

Lunges target the following muscles:

abdominals

back muscles

gluteal muscles

quadriceps

hamstrings

calves

Lunges are simple, making them accessible to people who want to add them to part of a longer routine or do them for a few minutes at a time throughout the day. You must stay on track and be consistent to maintain your results over time.

If you do lunges regularly as part of a larger fitness routine, you'll notice results in terms of building muscle mass and shaping up your body. You'll likely feel the results before they are visible.

You may develop tight, toned, and stronger muscles and start to lower your body fat percentage within a few weeks. More noticeable results may take a few months to develop.

For each lunge variation, do 2 to 3 sets of 8 to 12 repetitions. If you feel yourself starting to plateau, up the intensity by doing more difficult variations, adding weights, or increasing the amount you do.

The bottom line

The physical benefits of doing lunges may extend into other areas of your life, giving you more strength and confidence. Get the form down correctly before you move on to more challenging variations, and modify as necessary.

Even if significant weight loss isn't your goal, you may find that your legs and core are more toned. Base your accomplishments on how you feel and remember to take the time to rest and appreciate your efforts.

Stand on your feet shoulder width apart. ? Take left leg forward and lower down bending left knee at 90°. Knee of right leg would be just above the ground . ? Come back to the original position and take right leg forward. Do lunges with alternative legs. (This is 01 repetition) ? Do required number of repetitions. ? Keep your back straight throughout the movement. (c) Single leg squat This can be done with help of a partner or by holding a fix object . Again, keep your back straight throughout the movement.

Upper Body Crunches, also known simply as ab crunches, are used by many celebrities during Harley Pasternack's 5-Factor workout. Upper Body Crunches work the rectus abdominus, or upper abs. Think "six pack" or even "eight pack." The upper body crunch is one of the most common ab exercises. It is becoming common to perform crunches on stability or Bosu balls. This is because of the added work your core has to do to maintain the exercise.

Harley Pasternack likes his clients to do upper body crunches on Mondays. This is the day you work the rectus abdominus. Then, during your second workout of the week you work your lateral obliques. The third workout uses Lower Body Crunches to work your lower rectus abdominus, or the lower area of the six pack. Finally, during your last workout of the week, you do Double Crunches to work the upper abs and lower abs.

There is a mental cue that Harley Pasternack wants you to have through this exercise. He says that when doing the Upper Body Crunches you want to:

SHORTEN THE DISTANCE BETWEEN YOUR STERNUM AND BELLY BUTTON ON THE WAY UP, AND SHORTEN IT ON THE WAY DOWN.

To perform Upper Body Crunches:

Lie on your back on a padded or comfortable surface.

With knees bent on the floor, and hands loosely placed behind your head, tuck your chin in toward your chest.

Exhale as you bring your rib cage toward your pelvis.

Inhale, and return to lying down starting position.

As shown in the video below, you can use a mat. Try not to cave your chin in, instead keeping your head lifted throughout the exercise.

Popular Upper Body Crunches Workouts

The Lady Gaga workout uses Upper Body Crunches.

The Megan Fox workout uses Upper Body Crunches.

The Halle Berry workout uses Upper Body Crunches.

During her abs workouts, Instagram sensation Jen Selter uses Ab Crunches.

The Katy Perry workout uses Upper Body Crunches.

The Jennifer Garner workout starts with reverse crunches then moves to these Standard Crunches. She then does bicycle crunches, side planks, and forearm planks.

The Eva Mendez workout uses Upper Body Crunches.

Chris Hemsworth used this exercise to build his core for Thor.

The crew of 300 performed sit-ups during the Gerard Butler workout.

The Audrina Patridge workout used Ab Crunches to gain definition in her abs.

The Jay-Z workout, and the Beyonce workout, both use the upper body crunch modification. In their modification, you touch your heels on each crunch.

The Sylvester Stallone Expendables workout uses crunches. Stallone says:

CRUNCHES ARE MUCH MORE EFFECTIVE THAN REGULAR SIT-UPS BECAUSE THEY SPECIFICALLY TARGET YOUR UPPER ABDOMINAL MUSCLES RATHER THAN YOUR HIP MUSCLES. IF YOU'RE NOT USED TO THEM, THEY CAN CAUSE SORENESS A DAY OR TWO LATER, BUT IT'S A "COOL" SORENESS. A BADGE OF HONOR.

TUCK YOUR KNEES INTO YOUR CHEST AND REACH FOR YOUR HEELS. KEEP YOUR FEET TOGETHER. MAKE SURE YOUR HEELS AR IN THE SAME LINE YOUR YOUR HANDS: PARALLEL TO THE GROUND.

Upper Body Crunches Safety:

Make sure that your core is doing the work. Some people will stress their neck, but this is the wrong approach. Make sure that you squeeze your ab muscles and use them to propel you upwards.

When you think about your upper abs, you're really thinking about the top half of a muscle group called the rectus abdominis (known as your "six-pack" muscles), which runs down the front of your core from your ribs to your pubic bone. (FYI: This muscle group actually contains eight segments, not just six...but who's counting?)

It's important to keep your entire core strong by doing a wide variety of exercises—from isometric moves like planks to spine-flexing classics like crunches. However, if you want to specifically target your upper abs, you can do that by focusing on movements that involve pulling your chest toward your pelvis—or vice-versa.

Though the exercises in this upper abs workout do work your entire core (it's all connected!), they'll especially fire up that top half of your rectus abdominis.

Time: 20–25 minutes

Equipment: mat, light weight (optional)

Good for: upper abs (rectus abdominis)

Instructions: For this workout, you'll complete three or four rounds of the following four circuits, which each consist of either three or four moves. Perform each exercise for 30 seconds, then immediately continue to the next exercise in the circuit. Once you've completed the circuit, rest for 15 to 30 seconds, then repeat either two or three more times. At the end of each circuit, rest for 60 seconds and proceed to the next circuit. Repeat until finished.

1Circuit 1: Sprinter Situp

Good for: Rectus abdominis, obliques

How to: Start lying on back with hands by sides and legs extended straight on floor. Explosively sit up, bringing right knee toward chest, right arm back, and left arm forward at 90-degree angles. Reverse the motion with control and repeat on the other side. That's one rep. Complete as many reps as possible in 30 seconds, then immediately continue to the next exercise in this circuit.

2Bicycle Crunch

Good for: Rectus abdominis

How to: Lie on back with hands behind head. Lift shoulder blades off mat, raise legs so knees are bent at 90 degrees, and gaze at thighs, keeping neck relaxed. This is your starting position. Engage abs and rotate right elbow toward left knee while extending right leg straight, lowering it as close to the floor as possible without resting it on mat. Return to start and repeat on the other side. That's one rep. Complete as many reps as possible in 30 seconds, then immediately continue to the next exercise in this circuit.

3Plank to Toe Touch

Good for: Rectus abdominis, obliques, transverse abdominis (inner core)

How to: Start in plank position. Engage lower abs and lift hips to pull body into an upside down "V" shape while reaching right hand back to touch left ankle. (Heels stay high the whole time.) Slowly return to start. Repeat on the opposite side. That's one rep.

Complete as many reps as possible in 30 seconds. Then, rest for 15 to 30 seconds and repeat entire circuit two or three more times. From there, rest for 60 seconds and proceed to the second circuit.

4Circuit 2: Toe Reach

Good for: Rectus abdominis

How to: Start by lying on back with legs extended into the air to form a 90-degree angle with body. Lift arms so fingers point toward toes, then, keeping lower back pressed into mat, raise shoulders off mat as if to touch toes, then lower back down to start. That's one rep. Complete as many reps as possible in 30 seconds, then immediately continue to the next exercise in this circuit.

Make this move more difficult by holding a light weight.

5V-Up

Good for: Rectus abdominis, transverse abdominis

How to: Start lying on back with legs extended and arms by sides, both on mat. In one movement, lift upper body, arms, and legs, coming to balance on tailbone, forming a "V" shape with body. Lower body back down. That's one rep. Complete as many reps as possible in 30 seconds, then immediately continue to the next exercise in this circuit.

Make this move more difficult by holding a light weight.

6Plank Knee-To-Nose

Good for: Rectus abdominis, obliques, transverse abdominis

How to: Start in high plank position with left foot lifted slightly up off floor. Exhale and pull left knee toward chest while rounding spine to bring nose toward knee. With control, reverse movement to return to plank position with left foot lifted. That's one rep.

Complete as many reps as possible in 30 seconds. Then, rest for 15 to 30 seconds and repeat entire circuit two or three more times. From there, rest for 60 seconds and proceed to the third circuit.

7Circuit 3: Crunches

Good for: Rectus abdominis

How to: Start on back with knees bent, feet flat on the floor, and hands behind head. Keeping lower back pressed into the mat and belly button pulled in, lift chest toward the ceiling until shoulder blades come off the mat. Lower down. That's one rep. Complete as many reps as possible in 30 seconds, then immediately continue to the next exercise in this circuit.

8Alternating Leg Lowers

Good for: Rectus abdominis, obliques, transverse abdominis

How to: Lie on back. Keep hands by hips with lower back pressed into the mat. Lift both legs up to point straight toward ceiling. This is your starting position. With feet flexed, slowly lower right leg down. Bring right leg back up, then repeat with left leg. That's one rep. Complete as many reps as possible in 30 seconds, then immediately continue to the next exercise in this circuit.

Make this move more difficult by extending arms up toward ceiling or straight back overhead.

9Inchworm

Good for: full body

How to: Start standing at back of mat with feet hip-width apart and arms by sides. Slowly bend over and touch the floor in front of feet with both hands. Keeping legs as straight as possible and core tight, walk hands forward into a plank position. Pause, then slowly reverse the movement to return to start. That's one rep. Complete as many reps as possible in 30 seconds. Then, rest for 15 to 30 seconds and repeat entire circuit two or three more times. From there, rest for 60 seconds and proceed to the final circuit.

10Circuit 4: Jackknife Pullover

Good for: Rectus abdominis, obliques, transverse abdominis, shoulders

How to: Start lying on back, holding a single dumbbell or light kettlebell in hands like a goblet with arms straight; bend legs and curl shoulder blades up off the floor in order to bring elbows and knees to touch in air over stomach. Lower back to mat and stretch arms overhead while extending legs and lower to hover a few inches above the floor. Return to start. That's one rep. Complete as many reps as possible in 30 seconds, then immediately continue to the next exercise in this circuit.

Make this move more difficult by increasing the weight used. Make it easier by removing the weight.

11Half Get-Up (Left Side)

Good for: full body

How to: Start by lying on back with left leg bent, foot on floor, right leg extended out straight, right arm straight on floor at 45-degree angle from body, palm down, and left arm bent with triceps on mat (option to hold weight in left hand). Press left arm straight up, palm facing in, and keep gaze on hand. Shift weight onto right hip and roll to the right, propping body up on right forearm. Then, push through palm to extend right arm to straight. Slowly reverse steps to return to start. That's one rep. Complete as many reps as possible in 30 seconds, then immediately continue to the next exercise in this circuit.

Make this move more difficult by increasing the weight used.

12Half Get-Up (Right Side)

Good for: full body

How to: Start by lying on back with right leg bent, foot on floor, left leg extended out straight, left arm straight on floor at 45-degree angle from body, pam down, and right arm bent with tricep on mat (option to hold weight in left hand). Press right arm straight up, palm facing in, and keep gaze on hand. Shift weight onto left hip and roll to the left, propping body up on left forearm. Then, push through palm to extend left arm to straight. Slowly reverse steps to return to start. That's one rep. Complete as many reps as possible in 30 seconds, then immediately continue to the next exercise in this circuit.

Make this move more difficult by increasing the weight used.

13Mountain Climbers

Good for: full body

How to: Start in high plank position. Keep shoulders over wrists and back flat while quickly driving left knee toward chest, returning it to start, and repeating with right knee. That's one rep. Complete as many reps as possible in 30 seconds. Then, rest for 15 to 30 seconds and repeat entire circuit two or three more times. Then you're done!

Areas worked – upper abdominals Technique ? Lie on your back. Fold your legs so that your feet are close to your hips. Hands folded across your chest . ? Curl your torso 5-6 inches above the ground (Peak) . ? Slowly come back to the original position . (This is one repletion) ? Do required number of repetitions. Don'ts ? Don't flatten your legs on the ground. That would put undue stress on your lower back. ? Don't do jerky movements. All movements should be rhythmic and smooth. Hints and Tips ? Hold weight plates on your chest to increase the load. ? You can place your legs on a chair or in air for complete immobilization of your lower body . 50 ? Cross your hands over your head behind your back to increase load . ? Exhale while going up and inhale while coming down. Variation ? Lie on your back. Keep your hands straight on the ground, palm down, close to your body. ? Slide your palms 4-5 inches forward on the ground and come back to the original position. 4. LOWER ABDOMINAL CRUNCHES Areas worked – lower abdominals Technique ? Lie on your back. Fold your legs so that your feet are close to you . ? Lift knees towards chest and slowly lower down to the original position . (This is 01 repetition). ? Do required number of repetitions. Don'ts ? Don't place your feet away from the hips. Greater the distance of feet from hips, greater will be the stress on lower back. ? Never hold your breath during movement. Hints and Tips ? For greater range of movement this exercise can be performed by placing hips on the edge of a bench or bed . ? Range of movement should be limited so that it does not hurt your lower back.

CHAPTER FIVE

How to stay fit forever: 25 tips to keep moving when life gets in the way

Can you carry on exercising when your motivation slips, the weather gets worse or your schedule becomes overwhelming? Experts and Guardian readers give their best advice

When it comes to exercise, we think about how to "get" fit. But often, starting out is not the problem. "The big problem is maintaining it," says Falko Sniehotta, a professor of behavioural medicine and health psychology at Newcastle University. The official UK guidelines say adults should do strength exercises, as well as 150 minutes of moderate activity, or 75 minutes of vigorous activity, every week. According to the Health Survey for England in 2016, 34% of men and 42% of women are not hitting the aerobic exercise targets, and even more – 69% and 77% respectively – are not doing enough strengthening activity. A report from the World Health Organization last week found that people in the UK were among the least active in the world, with 32% of men and 40% of women reporting inactivity. Meanwhile, obesity is adding to the chronic long-term diseases cited in Public Health England's analysis, which shows women in the UK are dying earlier than in most EU countries.

We all know we should be doing more, but how do we keep moving when our motivation slips, the weather takes a turn for the worse or life gets in the way? Try these 25 pieces of advice from experts and Guardian readers to keep you going.

1 Work out why, don't just work out

Our reasons for beginning to exercise are fundamental to whether we will keep it up, says Michelle Segar, the director of the University of

Michigan's Sport, Health and Activity Research and Policy Center. Too often "society promotes exercise and fitness by hooking into short-term motivation, guilt and shame". There is some evidence, she says, that younger people will go to the gym more if their reasons are appearance-based, but past our early 20s that doesn't fuel motivation much. Nor do vague or future goals help ("I want to get fit, I want to lose weight"). Segar, the author of No Sweat: How the Simple Science of Motivation Can Bring You a Lifetime of Fitness, says we will be more successful if we focus on immediate positive feelings such as stress reduction, increased energy and making friends. "The only way we are going to prioritise time to exercise is if it is going to deliver some kind of benefit that is truly compelling and valuable to our daily life," she says.

2 Get off to a slow start

The danger of the typical New Year resolutions approach to fitness, says personal trainer Matt Roberts, is that people "jump in and do everything – change their diet, start exercising, stop drinking and smoking – and within a couple of weeks they have lost motivation or got too tired. If you haven't been in shape, it's going to take time." He likes the trend towards high-intensity interval training (HIIT) and recommends people include some, "but to do that every day will be too intense for most people". Do it once (or twice, at most) a week, combined with slow jogs, swimming and fast walks – plus two or three rest days, at least for the first month. "That will give someone a chance of having recovery sessions alongside the high-intensity workouts."

3 You don't have to love it

It is helpful not to try to make yourself do things you actively dislike, says Segar, who advises thinking about the types of activities – roller-skating? Bike riding? – you liked as a child. But don't feel you have to really enjoy exercise. "A lot of people who stick with exercise say: 'I feel better when I do it.'" There are elements that probably will be enjoyable, though, such as the physical response of your body and the feeling of getting stronger, and the pleasure that comes with mastering a sport.

"For many people, the obvious choices aren't necessarily the ones they would enjoy," says Sniehotta, who is also the director of the National Institute for Health Research's policy research unit in behavioural science, "so they need to look outside them. It might be different sports or simple things, like sharing activities with other people."

4 Be kind to yourself

Individual motivation – or the lack of it – is only part of the bigger picture. Money, parenting demands or even where you live can all be stumbling blocks, says Sniehotta. Tiredness, depression, work stress or ill family members can all have an impact on physical activity. "If there is a lot of support around you, you will find it easier to maintain physical activity," he points out. "If you live in certain parts of the country, you might be more comfortable doing outdoor physical activity than in others. To conclude that people who don't get enough physical activity are just lacking motivation is problematic."

Segar suggests being realistic. "Skip the ideal of going to the gym five days a week. Be really analytical about work and family-related needs when starting, because if you set yourself up with goals that are too big, you will fail and you'll feel like a failure. At the end of a week, I always ask my clients to reflect on what worked and what didn't. Maybe fitting in a walk at lunch worked, but you didn't have the energy after work to do it."

5 Don't rely on willpower

"If you need willpower to do something, you don't really want to do it," says Segar. Instead, think about exercise "in terms of why we're doing it and what we want to get from physical activity. How can I benefit today? How do I feel when I move? How do I feel after I move?"

6 Find a purpose

Anything that allows you to exercise while ticking off other goals will help, says Sniehotta. "It provides you with more gratification, and the costs of not doing it are higher." For instance, walking or cycling to work, or making friends by joining a sports club, or running with a friend. "Or the goal is to spend more time in the countryside, and running helps you do that."

Try to combine physical activity with something else. "For example, in my workplace I don't use the lift and I try to reduce email, so when it's possible I walk over to people," says Sniehotta. "Over the course of the day, I walk to work, I move a lot in the building and I actually get about 15,000 steps. Try to make physical activity hit as many meaningful targets as you can."

7 Make it a habit

When you take up running, it can be tiring just getting out of the door – where are your shoes? Your water bottle? What route are you going to take? After a while, points out Sniehottta, "there are no longer costs associated with the activity". Doing physical activity regularly and planning for it "helps make it a sustainable behaviour". Missing sessions doesn't.

8 Plan and prioritise

What if you don't have time to exercise? For many people, working two jobs or with extensive caring responsibilities, this can undoubtedly be true, but is it genuinely true for you? It might be a question of priorities, says Sniehotta. He recommends planning: "The first is 'action planning', where you plan where, when and how you are going to do it and you try to stick with it." The second type is 'coping planning': "anticipating things that can get in the way and putting a plan into place for how to get motivated again". Segar adds: "Most people don't give themselves permission to prioritise self-care behaviours like exercise."

9 Keep it short and sharp

A workout doesn't have to take an hour, says Roberts. "A well-structured 15-minute workout can be really effective if you really are pressed for time." As for regular, longer sessions, he says: "You tell yourself you're going to make time and change your schedule accordingly."

10 If it doesn't work, change it

It rains for a week, you don't go running once and then you feel guilty. "It's a combination of emotion and lack of confidence that brings us to the point where, if people fail a few times, they think it's a failure of the entire project," says Sniehotta. Remember it's possible to get back on track.

If previous exercise regimes haven't worked, don't beat yourself up or try them again – just try something else, he says. "We tend to be in the mindset that if you can't lose weight, you blame it on yourself. However, if you could change that to: 'This method doesn't work for me, let's try something different,' there is a chance it will be better for you and it prevents you having to blame yourself, which is not helpful."

11 Add resistance and balance training as you get older

"We start to lose muscle mass over the age of around 30," says Hollie Grant, a personal training and pilates instructor, and the owner of PilatesPT. Resistance training (using body weight, such as press-ups, or equipment, such as resistance bands) is important, she says: "It is going to help keep muscle mass or at least slow down the loss. There needs to be some form of aerobic exercise, too, and we would also recommend people start adding balance challenges because our balance is affected as we get older."

12 Up the ante

"If you do 5k runs and you don't know if you should push faster or go further, rate your exertion from one to 10," says Grant. "As you see those numbers go down, that's when to start pushing yourself a bit faster." Roberts says that, with regular exercise, you should be seeing progress over a two-week period and pushing yourself if you feel it is getting easier. "You're looking for a change in your speed or endurance or strength."

13 Work out from home

You don't need complex equipment. Illustration: Mark Long

If you have caring responsibilities, Roberts says you can do a lot within a small area at home. "In a living room, it is easy to do a routine where you might alternate between doing a leg exercise and an arm exercise," he says. "It's called Peripheral Heart Action training. Doing six or eight exercises, this effect of going between the upper and lower body produces a pretty strong metabolism lift and cardiovascular workout." Try squats, half press-ups, lunges, tricep dips and glute raises. "You're raising your heart rate, working your muscles and having a good general workout." These take no more than 15-20 minutes and only require a chair for the tricep dips – although dumbbells can be helpful, too.

14 Get out of breath

We are often told that housework and gardening can contribute to our weekly exercise targets, but is it that simple? "The measure really is you're getting generally hot, out of breath, and you're working at a level where, if you have a conversation with somebody while you're doing it, you're puffing a bit," says Roberts. "With gardening, you'd have to be doing the heavier gardening – digging – not just weeding. If you're walking the dog, you can make it into a genuine exercise session – run with the dog, or find a route that includes some hills."

15 Be sensible about illness

Joslyn Thompson Rule, a personal trainer, says: "The general rule is if it's above the neck – a headache or a cold – while being mindful of how you're feeling, you are generally OK to do some sort of exercise. If it's below the neck – if you're having trouble breathing – rest. The key thing is to be sensible. If you were planning on doing a high-intensity workout, you would take the pace down, but sometimes just moving can make you feel better." After recovering from an illness, she says, trust your instincts. "You don't want to go straight back into training four times a week. You might want to do the same number of sessions but make them shorter, or do fewer."

16 Seek advice after injury

Clearly, how quickly you start exercising again depends on the type of injury, and you should seek advice from your doctor. Psychologically, though, says Thompson Rule: "Even when we're doing everything as we should, there are still dips in the road. It's not going to be a linear progression of getting better."

17 Take it slowly after pregnancy

Again, says Thompson Rule, listen to your body – and your doctor's advice at your six-week postnatal checkup. After a caesarean section, getting back to exercise will be slower, while pregnancy-related back injuries and problems with abdominal muscles all affect how soon you can get back to training, and may require physiotherapy. "Once you're walking and have a bit more energy, depending on where you were before (some women never trained before pregnancy), starting a regime after a baby is quite something to undertake," says Thompson Rule. "Be patient. I get more emails from women asking when they're going to get their stomachs flat again than anything. Relax, take care of yourself and take care of your baby. When you're feeling a bit more energised, slowly get back into your routine." She recommends starting with "very basic stuff like walking and carrying your baby [in a sling]".

18 Tech can help

For goal-oriented people, Grant says, it can be useful to monitor progress closely, but "allow some flexibility in your goals. You might have had a stressful day at work, go out for a run and not do it as quickly and then think: 'I'm just not going to bother any more.'" However, "It can start to get a bit addictive, and then you don't listen to your body and you're more at risk of injury."

19 Winter is not an excuse

"Winter is not necessarily a time to hibernate," says Thompson Rule. Be decisive, put your trainers by the door and try not to think about the cold/ drizzle/greyness. "It's the same with going to the gym – it's that voice in our head that make us feel like it's a hassle, but once you're there, you think: 'Why was I procrastinating about that for so long?'"

READERS' TIPS

20 Keep it bite-size

Alex Tomlin

I've tried and failed a few times to establish a consistent running routine, but that was because I kept pushing myself too hard. Just because I can run for an hour doesn't mean I should. Running two or three times a week for 20-30 minutes each time has improved my fitness hugely and made it easier to fit in.

21 Reward yourself

Neil Richardson

I keep a large bag of Midget Gems in my car to motivate myself to get to the gym, allowing myself a handful before a workout. Sometimes I toss in some wine gums for the element of surprise.

22 Call in the reinforcements

Niall O'Brien

I tapped into the vast network of fitness podcasts and online communities. On days I lacked drive, I would listen to a fitness podcast, and by the time I got home, I would be absolutely determined to make the right choices. In fact, I would be excited by it. Your brain responds very well to repetition and reinforcement, so once you have made the difficult initial change, it becomes much easier over time.

23 Use visual motivation

Siobhan King

I have kept a "star chart" on my calendar for the past two years, after having three years of being chronically unfit. I put a gold star on days that I exercise, and it's a good visual motivator for when I am feeling slug-like. I run, use our home cross-trainer and do a ski fitness programme from an app. My improved core strength has helped my running and ability to carry my disabled child when needed.

24 Keep alarms out of reach

Sally Crowe

If, like me, you need to get up early to exercise or it just doesn't happen, move your alarm clock away from your bed and next to your kit. Once you have got up to turn it off, you might as well keep going!

25 Follow the four-day rule

Joanne Chalmers

I have one simple rule which could apply to any fitness activity – I do not allow more than four days to elapse between sessions. So, if I know I have a busy couple of days coming up, I make sure I run before them so that I have "banked" my four days. With the exception of illness, injury or family emergencies, I have stuck to this rule for 10 years.

CHAPTER SIX

No Gym Required: How to Get Fit at Home Get in shape without leaving the house

You want to get fit. But you don't want to join a health club -- it's too expensive, there's no gym convenient to you, or maybe you're just the independent type. Or perhaps you're already a gym member, but your schedule has been too manic for you to get away.

That leaves working out at home. But can you really get a great workout without leaving the house?

Absolutely, says Kevin Steele, PhD, exercise physiologist and vice president of 24 Hour Fitness Centers.

"In today's world, the reality of it is people don't have time to go to a facility every day anyway," he says. "And consistency is key."

Believe it or not, Steele says, at 24 Hour Fitness, they encourage folks to exercise at home as much as at the gym. This way, they are more apt to adopt fitness as a lifestyle. "The key thing is that you do something, somewhere, sometime," he says.

Steele and other fitness experts say it doesn't take much effort or money to design an effective workout program at home. Things like fit balls, dumbbells, exercise bands or tubing, and push-up bars are an inexpensive way to create a routine that works all the major muscle groups.

But even with no props or machines, you can build muscles and burn calories.

"If someone wants to get started, they could take a brisk walk, then do abdominal exercises and push-ups," says Richard Weil, MEd, CDE an exercise physiologist and WebMD Weight Loss clinic consultant.

A warmup.

A cardiovascular (aerobic) workout.

Resistance (strength-building) exercises.

Flexibility moves.

A cooldown

A warm-up could be an easy walk outside or on a treadmill, or a slow pace on a stationary bike. For the cardiovascular portion, walk or pedal faster, do step aerobics with a video, or jump rope -- whatever you enjoy that gets your heart rate up.

The resistance portion can be as simple as squats, push-ups and abdominal crunches. Or you could work with small dumbbells, a weight bar, bands or tubing.

Increase your flexibility with floor stretches or yoga poses. And your cooldown should be similar to the warm up, says Steele -- "cardiovascular work at a low level to bring the heart rate down to a resting state."

You can do strength work in same workout as your aerobic work, or split them up. Just be sure to warm up and cool down every time you exercise.

If you're short on time one day, increase the intensity of your workout, says Tony Swain, MS, fitness director of East Bank Club in Chicago. Instead of your usual 45-minute ride on the stationary bike, choose a harder program for 25 minutes and really push yourself. Choose the hilly walk in your neighborhood, or jog instead of walking.

You can step up the pace of your strength workout by doing compound exercises -- those that work more than one muscle group at a time.

For example, doing squats (with or without weights) works the quadriceps, hamstrings, gluteus, and calves. Push-ups involve the pectorals, deltoids, biceps, triceps -- even the abdominals and the upper back.

If you're not the create-your-own workout type, there are fitness videos galore -- offering everything from kickboxing to belly dancing to Pilates. You can find them at local bookstores and discount stores, or on the Web. Just be sure to choose one that's appropriate for your fitness level.

Getting Started

If you're a beginner, aim for 30 minutes of cardiovascular exercise at least three times a week, and 20 to 30 minutes of strength work three times a week. Be sure your strength workout covers all major muscle groups, in your upper body, lower body, abdominals and back. Shoot for three sets of 10-15 repetitions of each strength exercise.

No matter what type of exercise you do, be sure to start slowly and gradually increase your workout time and intensity. And don't forget to listen to your body, says Weil.

"Focus on the muscles that you think you should be working," he says. "See if you feel it there. If you're working your abs and you feel it in your neck, then it's not right. Close your eyes and start to tune in to your body."

Going to the gym isn't always the best option when you want to work out. In fact, sometimes it just doesn't make sense at all. Hitting the gym can be costly; both for your bank account and your precious free-time.

Personal trainers can get expensive, and even basic gym memberships can easily amount to hundreds of dollars a year. For those who are fortunate enough to be able to pay for professional assistance, PT's are great and can definitely be worth the money, but there are many ways to get fit for much less!

Getting to the gym can also cut into your time. It can take several hours a week to get to and from the gym, especially if you tend to go doing rush-hour. And wouldn't it be great to have the option to just work out in the convenience of your home?

If you're trying to save time and money, or you're simply more comfortable working out at home, get fit without a gym by using these tips:

Take advantage of free workout videos. These routines give you a lot of flexibility, as you can do them virtually anywhere, without equipment or a gym.

Walk when possible. Walking is the MOST underrated exercise. Going for a Sunday coffee? Save some gas money by going for a walk. You can also add extra steps to your day by parking further away to walk or by walking around when on the phone. Want to make it fun? Turn walking into a fun social event by inviting your friends or co-workers along for a Monday Mile.

Take the stairs. Elevators are great when you're going to the 10th floor, but taking the stairs whenever it's possible can make a big difference on your health. You can even walk up and down the stairs of your own house or apartment building to add a bit of exercise to your day. Did you know that climbing stairs burns more calories per minute than jogging?

Get your hands on some basic fitness equipment. Light dumbbells, a stability ball and jump rope can all be used for a great home-workout. If you can't afford equipment, ask family or friends if they have any workout equipment lying around that they're not using.

Get creative. This can actually get really fun. Think of items around the house that weigh more than a pound, but are easy to hold on to. Use them as weights by doing curls or squats. You can also use furniture as exercise equipment; try box squats or step ups on chairs. Get more ideas from these mini workouts!

Do bodyweight exercises. Planks, push-ups, squats, jumping jacks and step-ups are all great ways to get moving!

Make housework exercise time. Cleaning the house is actually a great way to get moving. Check out how many calories you can burn by doing housework with this calculator.

Did you wish for some fancy gym equipment for Christmas but didn't quite get what you wanted? If you didn't get a fancy treadmill, smart fitness mirror, smart boxing setup, digital weight machine, coveted exercise bike or one of the other buzzy fitness products out there, but still want to get in shape at home, good news. As helpful all of these products can be, you don't need them to get in shape. There's one tool that you already have that's seriously underrated: your own body.

Even though nice fitness gear, smart gyms, and equipment are great -- you really don't need any fancy dumbbells, or anything else for that matter, to get a great workout. In fact, using your own body weight is one of the best ways to get in shape.

I mean, think about it -- your body is pretty heavy. Being able to do a push-up, or pull up is pretty impressive in itself. And you don't have to buy anything or rely on any equipment to help you get strong, which is perfect when you don't have time to hit the gym, or you're far away from your home set up.

REASONS TO WORKOUT AT HOME

Let's face it, there are times when we just can't get to the gym for a workout. Maybe you have a little one at home, or have a tight schedule. Maybe you simply don't want to deal with a busy gym and having to fight the crowds that always seem to grow as the colder weather moves in and the New Year's resolution fitness crowd invades.
Sounds like the perfect opportunity to workout at home and get fit in the comfort of your home gym.
While some may struggle with adhering to working out at home, others are able to thrive and find they can take their workout routines to a whole new level.
Let's take a look the benefits of having your own home gym:

You'll Save Money

Depending on how much equipment you'll need, working out at home should be a big money saver over the long haul. Many gyms not only require a monthly membership fee, but they also have additional costs for things such as group classes and personal training.

With the popularity of bodyweight-only workouts, all you need is a little space and you can essentially workout for free! Many at-home exercise enthusiasts like to add some multi-purpose equipment like dumbbells, resistance bands, a yoga/stretching mat, or kettle bells. You can also pair those along with a cardio piece such as a treadmill, an elliptical, a bike, or a rower. While there's obviously an initial cost for equipment like this, over time it will be cheaper than paying for a membership where you're essentially renting equipment.

Time Saver

Not only can you choose workouts that best fit your schedule, you will also save time driving to and from the gym, checking in, changing in the locker room, waiting for equipment, etc. All of that often adds up to more time than your actual workout!

You can literally roll out of bed and workout and have plenty of time for a good post-workout meal before you start your day. You could come home after work, grab a workout, and enjoy a dinner at home before relaxing for the evening. If you're a stay-at-home parent or work from home, being able to grab a workout when you can is a huge bonus!

No Crowds

While most commercial gyms offer a nice variety of equipment, there's also often a bunch of others who want to use it too. The winter months tend to be more crowded. If you're a peak-time exerciser, not only will you fight the crowds in the gym, but you'll often have to deal with them in the parking lot and in the locker room.

Remember, gyms want (and need) to sell memberships, so if you're not willing to deal with the potential crowds that can come along with your gym visits, than a home gym may be a much better fit for you.

Focus on Your Workout

There can be a lot of distractions at the gym. Everything from people wanting to chat to the "can you give me a spot" guy. Finding a spot in the gym to zone out and focus shouldn't be harder than the workout itself.

At home, no one should disturb you so you should be able to better focus on your workout routine and benefit from a more productive workout.

You Pick The Music

Music can be a very motivating factor when working out, and being at home allows you to listen to whatever you want and at the volume you want. And you don't have to wear those annoying earbuds that keep wanting to fall out!

You can even work out your core a little by belting out songs. Keep it light and fun!

Wear What You Want

We all know that fitness should be more important than looks, but the days that you don't want to see anyone shouldn't keep you from working out! At home, no one is going to care that you're wearing last night's t-shirt and some dirty sweatpants to work out. The only thing you have to worry about is getting some sweat on your brow.

Working out at home allows you to wear whatever you want without being judged, stared at, or ridiculed.

Less Germs

There's nothing worse than going to your favorite piece of equipment at the gym only to find the previous user left you a nice puddle of sweat. Commercial gyms are filled with germs, from the cardio equipment to the benches to the weights.

At home, you at least know who has used the equipment and can control how clean you keep it.

If you're a regular gym goer, then that's great and you should keep it up! But, if going to the gym is a huge barrier to your fitness, consider starting a home gym. Cater it to your needs and start off small so that you're encouraged to use it.

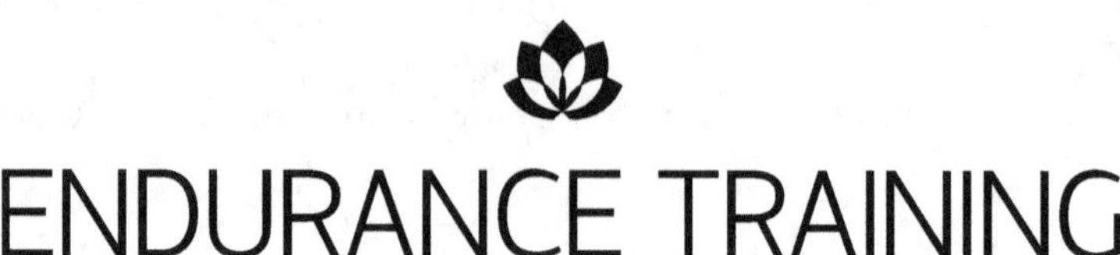

CHAPTER SEVEN

ENDURANCE TRAINING

Endurance exercise is an activity that increases your heart rate and breath for an extended period. To endure is to remain persistent and overcome challenges. It means moving forward when things are hard. Endurance exercise requires the same level of focus and dedication. This form of training is beneficial to your health.

To benefit from endurance exercise, you must know what it is and what effects it has. You must know how to integrate it into your training regimen. You must also be sure that you understand the importance of rest and how it affects your results. Applying this information will help you increase your base fitness level.

Read on to learn more about endurance exercise and how it can complement your training at Gloveworx.

Aerobic and Anaerobic Energy Systems

Your body is fueled by different energy systems that make your body move. For our purposes, we'll keep things very basic. There are two general types of energy systems in our bodies: aerobic and anaerobic.

Anaerobic Exercises

Anaerobic exercises are high-intensity workouts. During this type of activity the demand for oxygen exceeds the available supply. Simply put, anaerobic exercises consist of high performance for short bursts of time. Exercises like sprinting and heavy weight lifting are anaerobic.

Aerobic Exercises

Endurance exercise uses the aerobic energy system. During aerobic exercise, our oxygen consumption balances with our oxygen production. The lower oxygen consumption doesn't mean the exercise will be easy. Running a marathon is an aerobic exercise, but it's still 26.2 miles.

It's All Relative

It's important to keep in mind that people are at different levels. People have different aerobic and anaerobic thresholds. High-intensity and steady-state will have different meanings for everyone. Five minutes of cycling may tip a newcomer into an anaerobic state. On the other hand, it may be a nice warm up for a seasoned cyclist. As your body changes so will your metabolic rate. This will also change your reaction to physical activity.

The Benefits of Endurance Exercise

Aerobic exercises offer plenty of benefits. Some of these benefits come in the form of preventative medicine. Others benefit your training goals. Here are a few reasons why you should add endurance training to your program:

Fight Against Heart Disease

Endurance exercise causes a significant reduction in blood pressure and risk for heart disease. According to the American Heart Association, heart disease can include:

hypertension;

stenosis;

arrhythmias;

heart attacks;

strokes;

aneurysms;

congestive heart failure.

In addition to meeting your goals, you can take pride in the work you're doing to prevent serious health issues.

Improve Mental Clarity

When faced with long days at work and the endless duties of home life, it's normal to feel sluggish and unfocused. Aerobic exercises increase cognitive function. This special study was conducted on the elderly. The results show that aerobic exercise can offset the effects of aging. With aerobic exercise, you can get the focus you need to tackle your training and Become Unstoppable.

Build Your Oxygen Base

Oxygen is what fuels our muscles during physical activity. As intensity increases, so does our need for oxygen. Endurance exercises can help increase your oxygen capacity. This makes your body more efficient during exercise. As your body becomes more efficient, you can add to your routine. In time, your performance will improve. As such, adding endurance exercise to your program can help you build a foundation for the rest of your training.

Types of Endurance Exercise

Endurance exercise can be almost any form of steady physical activity. Essentially, it gets your blood flowing and increases your heart rate for a sustained period of time. Examples of endurance exercises include:

Walking

Running or jogging at a steady pace

Dancing

Cycling at a steady pace

Various sports

Bodyweight exercises such as squats, push-ups, sit-ups, lunges, etc.

Jump Rope/ Skipping

Swimming

Some of these exercises could also be classified as anaerobic. Sprinting, either in cycling or running, would be anaerobic. Try to find a challenging pace that you can maintain for at least ten minutes to start. You should be breathing heavily and sweating, but able to speak. Remember, intensity is relative to your fitness level. As you get stronger, your pace and stamina will progress.

HIIT Exercises

High-Intensity Interval Training, or HIIT, combines intense anaerobic bursts with periods of rest. Sometimes the rest periods include light aerobic exercises. High-intensity exercise has a proven effect on skeletal muscle function. This leads to an improved metabolism, strength, and level of endurance.

HIIT sessions combine the benefits of anaerobic and endurance training. Combining the two can optimize your results. The Gloveworx Signature Session uses HIIT methods to make contenders sweat! Ways to add HIIT to your training session include:

Alternate running or cycling at a steady pace with short burst sprints.

Adding resistance training (free weights, barbells, etc.) to your cardio session.

Circuit training with a mix of boxing and body weight exercises.

Remember, the better your oxygen uptake from endurance training, the better your HIIT workouts will be.

Why Rest is so Important

No matter what your preferred method of training is, rest days are a part of the program. Your Gloveworx coach can recommend how much rest is needed for your program. A lack of proper rest can result in injury, muscle-loss, and illness. When you exercise, you put your muscles through stress. Rest days allow your muscles to recover, so you can give it your all during your next training session.

Rest is essential with endurance exercise. Without proper nutrition, rest, and balance, endurance training can counteract muscle gain. In extreme cases, it can even cause muscle loss. This fact can deter athletes from adding endurance training to their program. Scheduling enough rest time in your plan will help you avoid these effects. Over-training is harmful, while balance is key.

Integrate Endurance Training with Gloveworx

Gloveworx coaches work with their contenders to help them achieve their goals. Your coach can add endurance training to your program for better health, focus, and results. With dedication, endurance training can create a solid fitness foundation. With time, you can build on this foundation to reach your goals.

As Gloveworx owner Leyon Azubuike said, "The sky is the limit and then some! And we're just getting started." It's time to find out how much you can endure!

Though there are various types of endurance training, e.g., walking, swimming, running, cycling, hiking etc., this chapter focuses only on running. Running is an excellent exercise for cardiovascular fitness. It hardly requires any equipment other than a good pair of shoes, some space and a will to run! We will discuss here both aerobic (endurance) and anaerobic (speed) running. The term aerobic literally means 'with oxygen'. During aerobic running there is enough oxygen available to your muscles. Therefore, you can run for hours, though at a slower speed. During running at high speed (anaerobic running) your body cannot meet the huge demand of oxygen to the muscles. Therefore, though you can run very fast, you cannot continue the activity for more than a few seconds. ENDURANCE RUNNING I. BENEFITS – There are many benefits of endurance running – (i) It is an excellent fat-burning exercise. When you run, initially your body depends more on carbohydrates and less on fats for energy. But after 30-35 minutes, the situation reverses and body starts burning more fats than carbohydrates for its energy need. (ii) It strengthens your cardiovascular system and protects against cardiovascular diseases. (iii) It increases the number and diameter of capillaries. Capillaries transport oxygen in and waste products out from muscle fibres. The end result of this is availability of more oxygen and more energy in your body system. 64 (iv) It increases the number and size of mitochondria. Mitochondria are microscopic structures inside your muscles. They are termed as 'power houses' or 'aerobic engines'. In the mitochondria carbohydrate, fat and protein break down in presence of oxygen and release energy. Therefore, bigger the size of mitochondria, the more energy will be generated for your longer, faster runs. This is one of the reasons, long distance runners go for slow long distance(SLD) runs to improve their performance. (v) Regular running develops a healthy 'addiction' among runners. There is an increase in the mental alertness, awareness of surroundings, effortlessness, feeling of well-being, and euphoric relaxation especially after 30-40 minutes of continuous run. This phenomenon is termed as 'runner's high' and is worth trying. (vi) Long distance running at low intensity is one of the most powerful anti-depressant 'natural' drugs. Try it yourself. Next time when you get anxious, angry or depressed, put on your shoes and jog for 30-40 minutes. Your depression will vanish. I have tried it on several occasions with definite success (though for me it requires at least one hour of jog). Students may practise it before their exams, or before appearing for an important interview. II. ENDURANCE RUNNING PROGRAMME DESIGN Your endurance running programme design will be guided by your specific goal. Let's discuss the FITT factors for running. A. Frequency – 3-5 days of endurance run per week produces reasonable cardiovascular fitness. The number of training days per week depends on the intensity (heart rate) and volume (duration) of training. For beginners and non-athletes 3 days of training on alternate days will be sufficient. Athletes may train on 5-6 days with 1-2 days of rest. However, they have to alternate their training days as 'hard' and 'easy'. Hard days will be marked by 65 high intensity / high volume. Easy days will be marked by low intensity / low volume. Some studies suggest that one can maintain his aerobic fitness by training only 2 days per week, but for that your intensity/volume has to be on higher side. B. Intensity – Intensity is the most important factor in endurance run programme design and hence it deserves a detailed discussion. In simple words, intensity in running is related to how hard you run. The 'hardness' or intensity, is measured by heart rate BPM (beats per minute). At increased intensity the heart rate also increases. Let's first understand these terms – Maximum Heart Rate (MHR), Resting Heart Rate(RHR), Training Heart Rate (THR) and Heart Rate Reserve (HRR). MHR is the maximum safe limit of heart rate for exercise. It is determined by subtracting one's age from 220. If some woman is 30, her MHR will be 220-30=190 BPM (beat per minute). RHR is the heart rate taken when you are fully rested and relaxed. The best time to take RHR is immediately after you wake up in the morning, while still lying in bed. HRR is the number beats per minute (BPM) that the heart rate can increase from resting up to the maximal. How to determine Training Heart Rate (THR)? It is important to determine the required intensity (required heart rate) of your training to reach your fitness goal. There are two methods to determine THR – (i) % MHR method and (ii) % HRR method. (i) % MHR method – MHR is determined by subtracting one's age from 220. Thus, for a 30 year old person MHR will be 220-30 =190 BPM (beat per minute). For a generally healthy person Training Heart Rate (THR) for aerobic fitness will be in the range of 70%-85% of MHR. (In this example, minimum and maximum THR for 30 year old will be (70% x 190=) 133 66 and (85% x 190=) 161.5 (say 162) BPM.) For those whose aerobic fitness level is very poor, a lower range of 55-65% of MHR may be more appropriate1 . Though % MHR method is a simple method, it has its own limitations. It does not take into account the existing aerobic fitness level of a person and prescribes the same THR to all persons of the same age. This method ignores the fact that in case of persons with higher fitness level, the training intensity has to be higher for their further gain. For example, exercising at 60% of MHR can benefit a sedentary person of 30, but an athlete of the same age is hardly going to gain anything at 60% of MHR. It will be a total waste of time for him. Therefore, THR by % MHR method should not be used blindly in all cases. THR with a higher % is recommended for those who have higher fitness level. For example, a fit person can have 70% or 80% MHR as his THR. (ii) % HRR method – This method, though apparently complicated, is more accurate in prescribing THR. It is based on the Karvonen formula. It takes into account the existing aerobic fitness level of a person. In this method there are two steps – Step-1. HRR=MHR–RHR Step-2. THR=(HRR x exercise intensity) + RHR If your age is 30, your RHR is 70, and you have to train at 60% intensity of HRR, Calculate your THR thus – Step-1. HRR = MHR – RHR = (220-30) BPM – 70 BPM = 120 BPM Step-2. THR = (HRR x intensity) + RHR = (120 x 60%) BPM + 70 BPM = 142 BPM

The recommended THR for aerobic fitness by % HRR method is 50- 85% of HRR2 . Why is it useful to take RHR into account while determining THR? Because, RHR is an important indicator of one's aerobic fitness. As one becomes more fit, his RHR decreases. Normally, a healthy person's

RHR will be 60-80 BPM. Endurance athletes often have their RHR below 60 BPM. (The famous cyclist, Lance Armstrong who won Tour de France consecutive seven record times, has RHR around 32 BPM3 .) And, as the RHR decreases, one's HRR will increase. This means that he can train himself at greater intensity. A. Technique of taking heart rate – You can take your heart rate by placing finger on carotid artery (located on both sides of the Adam's apple), or on radial artery (wrist) or simply by placing hand over your heart. Ideally, Training heart rate should be taken still while running. But as it is inconvenient to do so by above mentioned methods, the second best option is to take heart rate immediately after running. Take pulse count for 06 seconds and then multiply it by 10 to get your heart rate per minute. Or, you can take pulse count for 10 seconds and multiply it by 06 to get heart rate per minute. Alternatively, if you can afford, buy a good heart rate monitor and monitor your heart rate while running. Take heart. It is not necessary to take your heart rate in each running session. After monitoring your heart rate for some time, you may get a fair idea of your intensity level based on your biofeedback/exertion level. Important – It is important to avoid 'too soon too much' approach while determining your THR. Train at the THR that you can maintain throughout a 20- 30 minute running session. If you are running at THR based on 80% of your HRR and have to slow down or stop after 5-10 minutes, this means that you are overexerting yourself. Lower the % HRR down to 70% or 60% at which you can run comfortably all through the session. Running at unreasonably high THR is counterproductive and entails risk of injury also. One simple way to measure intensity while running is the 'talk test'. If you get so much breathless during running that you cannot talk to your partner, the intensity is too high for you. Slow down a bit so that you can talk to your partner comfortably. B. Time – How long one should run? Well, it depends on what is your goal. Generally, one should run for at least 20-30 minutes for cardiovascular fitness. If you are a long distance runner, run as per your training schedule which may extend to hours together. Training for distance runs (cross country, marathons, ultramarathons) is a specialized training and one should take help of professional coaches and books on these sports. C. Type – For cardiovascular fitness other alternatives to running are – brisk walk, rope skipping, swimming , cycling, rowing, hiking, stair climbing, any activity that engages you continuously for at least 20-30 minutes at an increased heart rate. III. OTHER IMPORTANT POINTS (i) Total weekly training volume (total number of kms run every week) should not be increased by more than 10% (to avoid overtraining) 4 . (ii) If you discontinue training, your fitness gains will reduce by approximately 50% within 4-12 weeks5 . Galloway, based on his experience, observes that you hardly lose conditioning within first five days of complete rest. However, for each week thereafter you will lose 25% of your fitness level. Thus after complete rest for a month, you will have to start like a 'beginner'. He suggest a rule of thumb i.e., in case of complete rest you'll need at least twice the number of weeks you took off to gradually reach back the pre-off level of fitness6 . (iii) To introduce variety, you should 'cross train' by occasionally taking up swimming, cycling, etc. During cross training your running muscles get some rest but your cardiovascular fitness remains the same. This cross training should be of the same intensity and volume, then only it will maintain your cardiovascular fitness. (iv) If you don't have time (or energy) to carry on running session for 20- 30 minutes, you can do it in 10-minute bouts also, twice or thrice in a day. (v) In endurance running as you need lot of oxygen, you can breathe through both your nose and mouth partly open. Normally, we should breathe through our nose because our nostrils filter the air and adjust the temperature of incoming air to our body's temperature. Mouth does not have this mechanism. But as the volume of oxygen during long running cannot be sufficient through nose breathing alone, we advise to breathe through mouth also. (vi) Take sufficient carbohydrates within half an hour after training to compensate for calories lost during long running. In absence of sufficient carbohydrates body will utilize protein for energy and your muscles will suffer. (vii) If you are running for more than 40-50 minutes, take care to hydrate yourself regularly by sipping water. This becomes all the more important if you are running in a hot weather. (viii) Adopt proper form and technique of running – Keep yourself upright and relaxed throughout. Arms should be bent at the elbows and forearm should move loosely parallel to the ground at waist level. Don't clench your fists. Fists should be loose and wrists relaxed. Take natural strides. Don't let your foot land too far in front of your body (fig-49). It will have a 'braking' effect on your speed and will cause more stress on your knees. Ideally, foot should land under the hips (fig-50). Take rhythmic, relaxed steps. Avoid raising your steps too high in the air as it results in a harder landing and greater stress on lower back and leg joints. Keep your feet low to the ground to avoid harder landing. (ix) Preferably run on softer surfaces like dirt or grass rather than on roads. (x) Use good pair of shoes and socks for better shock absorption during running. Fig-49

Fig-50 IV. HOW TO TRAIN FOR BETTER PERFORMANCE? The following will help you to improve you long distance run performance – (i) Slow long distance (SLD) runs – SLD runs at low intensity (60- 70% of MHR) form the base of any long distance running training. Low intensity practically means such level of effort that does not 71 make you breathless at any point of time. SLD runs increase the number of capillaries and mitochondria which contribute to faster and longer runs. (See Benefits of Endurance Running). You should run SLD once every week (not more than this). The distance of SLD should be longer than distance of your target race (e.g., 5 km, 10 km, half marathon, marathon, etc.). For example, if your target is to race 5 km, your SLD should cover more than 5 kms. Galloway's suggestion is to run SLD of 10-12 miles if your goal is 5 km race, 16-18 miles for 10 km race, 17-19 miles for half marathon, and 28-30 miles for marathon7 . I remind that while aiming for the maximum SLD, progression principle of exercise should be kept in mind. You should not increase more than 1 km distance every week. (ii) Hill training – Hill training strengthens our legs (especially calves) and cardiovascular system by offering more resistance. The place for training can be a hill with gentle slope, or flyover or steps of stadium / stairs of a multistoried building. Hill training is hard training. It should be introduced in later part of the endurance run training only after body is sufficiently conditioned through easy SLD runs. Run up the hill at 80-90% HRR effort. Take care not to become breathless at any point of time. Relax by walking down the hill before each repetition of the hill run. The maximum duration of hill training should be 15-20 minutes. Warm up well by jogging for 10-15 minutes before doing hill training, as hill runs are very demanding. During hill runs run on your toes with slightly higher knees. Keep your body upright while running. (iii) Interval training – Interval training consists of speed runs with rest intervals between two speed runs. It can be done on tracks in segments of 100 m / 200 m / 400 m or even more distance. Run, for (iv) example, 100 mtrs, recover by jog or walk till your heart rate drops to 60% of MHR, then do the next repetition of 100 mtr, and so on. Interval training should be done at 80-90% HRR intensity and should be of 15-20 minutes duration. Jog for 10-15 minutes before starting interval training session. Interval training is very helpful in improving speed. (v) Weight training – Weight training for endurance run focuses more on muscular endurance rather than on muscular strength. Weight training gives all the benefits of strength training (see section on Strength Training) and increases overall fitness of an endurance runner. They should train themselves by doing 2-3 sets (each set of 12-15 repetitions) of exercises (for both upper body and lower body) with less recovery time between two sets. Weight training makes their running muscles stronger and contributes to faster speed. (vi) Walk breaks – Galloway advocates introducing frequent 'walk breaks' for improving performance in endurance run8 . Walk break may be approximately of 1 minute duration. The idea is to take walk break whenever you feel that your running intensity is getting higher than your target rate. Take walk break before you fully exhaust yourself. You can take several walk breaks during a race. In many cases, this technique has been found to improve the performance. V. EXERCISES TO IMPROVE ENDURANCE RUN PERFORMANCE For overall fitness – Upper and lower body exercises mentioned in sections on strength Training and Flexibility Training.

SPEED RUNNING Speed is any activity continuously performed at approximately 100% effort for about 6 seconds. Generally, this is the maximum duration of time a person will be able to hold his maximum speed in a race. This is the duration in which he would 'explode'. To be able to maintain the maximum speed beyond 6 seconds one requires a great deal of training. I. BENEFITS (i) Speed helps in almost all track and field sports and games. It is especially beneficial to school children to excel in school sports and games. (ii) It helps strengthen our fast-twitch muscle fibres and thus improves speed element in endurance runs also. Speed training is an essential element in all endurance run training programmes. II. SPEED RUNNING PROGRAMME DESIGN A. Frequency – It depends upon your specific goal. Speed training is hard training and requires sufficient recovery time between two repetitions / sets. For a person training mainly for speed, the frequency may be 3-4 days per week; for endurance runners 1-2 days; for a normal person also 1-2 days. B. Intensity – Speed training is done at very high intensity. Therefore, before starting next repetition or next set one should recover well by slow jog, walk and stretch to bring his heart rate to almost normal level. The number of repetitions or sets should be increased gradually every week. Be careful. 'Too much too soon' approach will invite injury only. 81 C. Time – The actual time on speed training will depend upon the number of repetitions and sets in a training session. However, since it is a hard training, total duration should not exceed 20-30 minutes. Each speed training session should start with sufficient warm-up by 10-15 minutes of jog and stretch and should be concluded with proper cool-down. Failing to warm up and cool down will make your muscles stiff and susceptible to injury. D. Type – There is no alternative to speed running. To excel in speed run, you have to run at speed. That's all. III. OTHER IMPORTANT POINTS (i) Master the correct technique and form of speed running. The technique of speed running is different from that of endurance running in the following aspects – a) For speed, you push and land on the ball of the foot, not on the heel or flat foot as in endurance run. b) The correct technique for a good sprint start is to start at 45? angle and then quickly move upright throughout the race (fig63) 82 c) High knee lift (when thigh becomes parallel to the ground) combined with good stride length is correct technique of speed running. In endurance running, knees are not lifted to this degree. Here also, like endurance running technique, one should take care not to place foot far ahead of the body, but to place it directly under the hips.

(ii) Speed running is done not only by legs, but also by arms. The more aggressive your arms action forward and backward, the more will be your speed. Arms should be flexed to 90? and move forward and backward (maintaining the same elbow angle) almost parallel to the ground

(iii) If you have to train for both speed and endurance, do it on two different days. It you have to do both on the same day, do it in two different sessions (one in the morning and the other in the afternoon). If you have to do both in the same session, complete speed training first, recover and then start endurance training. (iv) You cannot achieve your peak training potentiality in both speed and endurance run simultaneously. Speed run is primarily dependent on fast-twitch muscle fibres and endurance run on slow-twitch muscle fibres. Therefore, you have to select your specific goal (speed running or endurance running) and train accordingly.

(v) For overall fitness, like for armed forces personnel, students or a common person, good strategy to improve both speed and endurance will be to combine the both in this manner – for two months do endurance training on 3-4 days and speed training on 2 days; next two months do endurance training on 2 days and speed training on 3-4 days, and so on. This strategy will gradually bring improvement in both while maintaining the gains in both. IV. HOW TO TRAIN FOR BETTER PERFORMANCE? (i) Speed running is primarily based on strength. Therefore, to improve speed overall body strength training is recommended. A look at the sprinters' muscular body will make this point clear. (ii) Mimic running movements while standing. For example, take small weights in hand and do arm action as you would do while running; lift knees to 90?; (try to) kick your butt with your heels, etc. (iii) Do short sprints of 10-20 mtrs with adequate recovery in between. (iv) Wear tight shoes (in endurance training we recommended for slightly larger sized shoes) with good sole grips. (v) Do stretching exercise religiously.

Exercises to Improve Speed Running For overall strength and flexibility – exercises mentioned in sections on Strength Training and Flexibility. Speed run-specific exercises – 1. Butt kicking – ? Stand on your feet. 85 ? Keeping rest of the body stationary, kick your butts alternatively with both heels. Don't allow your thighs to move forward or backward. ? Do 30-40 repetitions with each heel. 2. Arm action – ? Stand on your feet. ? Hold light weight in each hand and swing your arms forward and backward simulating arm action during running. Arms should be bent at 90? at elbows throughout and upper arm will be parallel to the ground. Movement should be rhythmic. Fig-65 86 ? This can be done without weights also. 3. Stride frequency drill – ? Run short sprints focusing mainly on maximizing the number of strides in a given time. ? You can do it in a stationary position also. 4. Stride length drill – ? Run short sprints at low intensity focusing mainly on increasing the stride length. ? Never overdo the stride length as it may injure you. Do some stretching exercise especially for hamstrings and calves to avoid injury. V. SAFETY FACTORS (i) Do proper warm-up and cool-down before and after speed training session respectively. (ii) Keep the duration of session short. (iii) Keep your abdominal and lower back muscles strong to avoid any undue stress on you lower back. (iv) Speed training is mostly a safe training.

FLEXIBILITY TRAINING Flexibility refers to the range of movement or motion (ROM) of a joint (e.g., elbow) or a series of joints (e.g., spine). In other words, flexibility is the ability of a joint to move freely through its full normal range of motion. Good flexibility allows maximum ROM during our dayto-day work and improves our performance in exercise. It also prevents injury like muscle tears or low back pain. As we age, we experience a progressive loss of flexibility due to disease, deterioration of joint structures, etc. In combination with loss of strength, loss of flexibility plays a significant role in accidental falls-related injuries in advance age. Stiff muscles or stiff connective tissues restrict full ROM. There are two important things about flexibility training. Firstly, a flexibility training must address all primary joints or series of joints for overall flexibility. Unless this is done, it is quite possible that a person may have excellent flexibility in a certain joint and at the same time he may suffer from poor flexibility of some other joint. Secondly, it has been found that flexibility can be improved at any age by proper stretching exercises. Inclusion of flexibility training in warm-up and cool-down phases (though traditionally recommended) is now a matter of debate. Some authors are of the opinion that static stretching during warm-up phase may actually adversely affect the force-producing capabilities of muscles. This school of thought recommends that a warm-up session consisting of only cardio-respiratory exercise may be more effective in increasing flexibility than static stretching. However, in my opinion till the time this debate is settled, it is safer to include flexibility training during warm-up and cooldown process. 88 I. BENEFITS (i) Flexibility training prevents stiffness of joints and makes our day to day movements comfortable. (ii) It prevents injury during sudden or excessive movement of joints. For example, a person with less flexible spine is more likely to incur injury during sudden bend to catch a falling glass. (iii) It is very relaxing. Yogic stretching (Yogasanas) is far more beneficial than normal stretching. It improves not only ROM of joints, but also helps internal systems (nervous system, digestive system, etc.). II. FLEXIBILITY TRAINING PROGRAMME DESIGN A. Frequency ? It should be done preferably on every day. Discontinuity of flexibility training even for a week drastically reduces our flexibility. Secondly, briefly stretching a muscle immediately after completion of each set removes lactic acid and helps faster recovery. For example, after completing a set of push ups, immediately stretch your pectoral muscles for faster recovery; or, stretch your quadriceps and hamstrings immediately after each set of squats, and so on. B. Intensity ? Stretching should be done to the point of slight discomfort but never to the point of pain. At least in matters of stretch, never compete with anyone. There would be sure chance of injury. C. Time ? Stretching during warm-up and cool-down may be for shorter duration (10-15 seconds each stretching). However, for improvement of flexibility, stretching should be for 30-60 seconds duration. During holding period of stretch one should breathe normally. Holding one's breath may cause dizziness. 89 D. Type ? There are mainly two types of flexibility training – (i) Active stretching – Hold a stretch at the extreme of ROM of a joint for 10-30 seconds. (ii) Passive stretching – Take assistance of partner or equipment (e.g., towel, rope) to reach you full ROM. Ballistic or bounce stretching is done to achieve greater ROM by using momentum of the body or bouncing. It is a very popular type of stretching in traditional physical training programmes. It is in fact flexibility and endurance training combined together. However, for not so well conditioned individuals it may be potentially dangerous as uncontrolled bouncing may cause injury. III. EXERCISES TO IMPROVE FLEXIBILITY 1. For neck – (i) • Sit (or stand) upright. ? Roll the head in a circle from left to right 2-3 times. ? Do the same from right to left. (ii)• Bring the chin down to touch your chest. Hold for 5-10 seconds. ? Lift your chin up and stretch your neck backward. Hold it for 5-10 seconds. (iii)• Bend your head over left shoulder. Hold it for 5-10 seconds. ? Bend your head over right shoulder. Hold it for 5-10 seconds. 2. For shoulders – (i) • Stand or sit upright. ? Position your hand on your shoulders . ? Rotate your elbows forward, 10 times. ? Rotate your elbows backward, 10 times.

(ii) •Extend the arms parallel to the ground. ? Rotate the shoulders forward and make a big circle with the arms 2-3 times ? Rotate the shoulders backward and make a big circle with the arms 2- 3 times.

3. For chest – ? Stand upright with your back against a window bar. Grip the bar at waist height. ? While gripping the bar, try to move away from the bar as far as possible fully extending your arms. Hold the stretch for 10 seconds. ? Keep your body upright throughout. ? This is good stretch for deltoids and biceps also.

4. For upper back – (i) • Stand or sit upright. ? Extend your arms at shoulder height, palms facing outward. Interlace your fingers ? Extend the arms and shoulders further forward till you feel stretch in upper back. Hold it for 10 seconds.

(ii)• Hold a window bar at shoulder height. ? Move away from the bar as far as possible (till you feel the stretch in your upper back). Hold it for 10 seconds. ? Keep your posture upright throughout.

5. For lower back – ? Do Bhujangasana as described under section on Yogic stretching. 6. For Quadriceps – ? Stand upright. ? Grip the ankle of left leg with right hand and pull it so that your left foot heel touches your right hip ? Hold it for 10-15 seconds. ? Do similar stretch with right leg with left hand.

7. For hamstrings – (i) Do Pashchinmottanasana. If you have problem in bending forward, do this – ? Sit down on floor extending right leg to the front closing left leg to your body . ? Grip the ball of the left foot with both hands and extend the left leg to the front as far as you can. ? Hold it for 10-15 seconds. ? Extend left leg to the front and close right leg to your body. ? Grip the ball of the right foot with both hands and extend the right leg to the front as far as possible. ? Hold it for 10-15 seconds.

8. For groins – ? Adopt lunging position with left foot forward and right leg straight. ? Lean forward to stretch the right groin muscles. Hold it for 10-15 seconds. ? Repeat the similar action with right foot forward and left leg straight to stretch left groin muscles.

9. For calves – (i) • Stand on the edge of a stair . ? Hold it for 10-15 seconds. (ii) • Lean against a wall with left foot forward and right leg extended ? Lean further keeping your back straight and right foot firmly planted to feel stretch in right calf. Hold it for 10-15 seconds. ? Keep the right heel on the ground throughout. ? Do similar action with right foot forward and left leg extended.

10. For ankles – ? Lean against the wall as described in stretching exercise number alternatively. ? Raise your heel slightly above the ground to stretch ankles. Yogic stretching 1. Pashchimotanasan ? This asana stretches almost whole body, particularly hamstrings, calves and small of the back. It improves digestion also. ? Sit erect. Stretch out legs. ? Bend forward and grasp your toes. ? Pull the toes towards yourself and rest your forehead on the knees. ? Maintain the stretch for 20-30 seconds. ? Come back to starting position.

Important ? Don't do this asana if you have lower back problem.

2. Bhujangasana – This is an excellent stretching for the back and whole spinal column. ? Lie on your abdomen, keeping arms close to your sides, palms beneath shoulders. ? Pushing the ground with your hands. Bend backward till your upper abdomen is up and navel still touching the ground. ? Maintain the stretch for 20-30 seconds. ? Come back to the starting position.

3. Dhanurasana – This is an excellent whole body stretching, especially for arms, shoulders, quadriceps and back. ? Lie on your abdomen. Bend the legs and grasps ankles. ? Pull the legs upward and simultaneously raise upper body. Aim to balance your body on the navel region. ? Maintain the stretch for 5-10 seconds. ? Come back to the starting position.

4. Gomukhasan – This is very good stretching of the upper back, shoulders and triceps. ? This can be done in traditional sitting position or even in upright sitting or standing position. ? Bring the left arm behind the back, palm facing outward, moving up along the spine. Push the forearm up as far as possible. Folding the right ear, palm facing inward, slide down the right hand forearm behind the back till the right hand touches the left hand. ? Aim to lock the forefinger of both hands together. ? Hold it for 10-15 seconds. ? Return to the original position.

IV. SAFETY FACTORS ? Preferably stretching should be done only towards the end of warmup. ? Stretch to the point of discomfort, but not pain. There will not be any gain from this pain. ? Never stretch an injured part. It will further aggravate the injury. ? Adopt correct form and technique. ? Breathe normally. ? All movements should be in rhythmic manner. ? Sometimes too much of flexibility may be too good to be desirable. Excessive flexibility may lead to injury especially in heavy weight lifting exercises.

Focus your mind on correct technique of movement. Try to do it better than the previous day. ? Don't do forward bending in case of any lower back problem.

Endurance training generally refers to training the aerobic system as reluctant to the anaerobic system. The Aerobic energy system uses fats, carbohydrates and proteins for re-synthesizing ATP (Adenosine triphosphate) for energy use. The Anaerobic System provides the body with explosive short term energy without the need for oxygen.

The need for endurance in sports is often asserted as the need of cardiovascular and simple muscular endurance, but the offspring of endurance is far more complex. Endurance is divided into two categories:-

General Endurance

Specific Endurance

General endurance symbolizes the ability of your whole body to tolerate endurance exercises and reduce fatigue. Whereas, Specific endurance symbolizes the ability to stand against tiredness in sport specific conditions. The better your sport specific endurance, the better you perform at this specific sport. And the better your general endurance the better you can stand longer efforts at your sport.

Endurance training is essential for a variety of endurance sports such as running, cycling, dancing, tennis, football, swimming, badminton, etc. Athletes also undergo endurance training when their sport is not necessarily an endurance sport in the whole sense but it demands some endurance.

Here are some Benefits of Endurance Training for Athletes:-

Endurance training can boost production of the hormones and helps increase metabolism.

Endurance training is effective at improving the heart's ability to pump oxygenated blood and reducing the risk of cardiovascular disease.

Reduces the symptoms of depression and boosts confidence and self-esteem.

It improves muscle mass and immunity of an athlete

Improves bone density and overall strength,

It improves mental health and sleep quality.

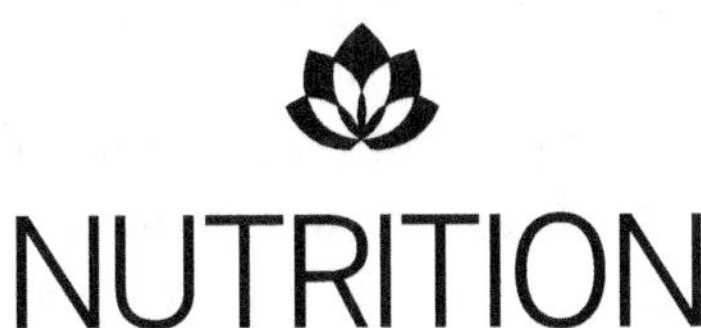

CHAPTER EIGHT

NUTRITION

Nutrition is a critical part of health and development. Better nutrition is related to improved infant, child and maternal health, stronger immune systems, safer pregnancy and childbirth, lower risk of non-communicable diseases (such as diabetes and cardiovascular disease), and longevity.

Healthy children learn better. People with adequate nutrition are more productive and can create opportunities to gradually break the cycles of poverty and hunger.

Malnutrition, in every form, presents significant threats to human health. Today the world faces a double burden of malnutrition that includes both undernutrition and overweight, especially in low- and middle-income countries.

WHO is providing scientific advice and decision-making tools that can help countries take action to address all forms of malnutrition to support health and wellbeing for all, at all ages.

This fact file explores the risks posed by all forms of malnutrition, starting from the earliest stages of development, and the responses that the health system can give directly and through its influence on other sectors, particularly the food system.

Proper nutrition in combination with adequate exercise and emotional well-being is the key to optimal performance of human mind and body. Lately, lot of research has been done in the field of dietetics. But all these studies have certain inherent limitations. One of the major limitations of these studies is that they have often been conducted on small groups of population or on rats in the laboratories. Even within the same group, different members have responded in different ways to dietary stimulus. For example, in many case studies, where the group was put on the same diet and exercise regimen, some of the group members gained weight, while the others did not gain any weight at all. However, despite all these limitations there are certain basic principles of nutrition which are supported by scientific research as well as by empirical findings. Preparation of diet plan is not a matter of plain arithmetics in which calculations are made on the basis of calories, proteins, carbohydrates, vitamins, etc. A balanced diet plan for an individual has to take into account several other important factors, e.g., age, gender, nature of physical and mental work, health status, sensitivity to a particular food, income, family food tradition etc. This section explains the basics of nutrition and provides broad guidelines for diet planning. Principles of nutrition There are three basic principles of nutrition:- i) Our body requires six essential nutrients, viz., proteins, carbohydrates, fats, vitamins, minerals and water. 106 ii) These nutrients are found in four basic food groups, viz., (a) cereals (b) vegetable/fruits, (c) meat/meat substitutes, (d) dairy products iii) The food items from these groups have to be consumed each day in the way that our maximum food intake comes from cereals followed by vegetables/ fruits, meat/meat-substitutes and dairy products. Food guide pyramid US Department of Agriculture (USDA) has developed the following food guide pyramid as guidelines for daily dietary intake from different food groups, which can be useful for us also. Serving size for different food groups Important – The number of servings given in the food pyramid is recommended for the entire day. For example, 4 slices of breads in the breakfast, ½ cup rice in the lunch, 4 chapatis in the dinner, ½ cup dal in the 1. Bread, cereal, rice 1 slice of bread, ½ cup of cooked cereal/rice (1 cup is equivalent to volume of a tennis ball/ approx. 8 tablespoons) 2. Vegetables ½ cup of cooked vegetable 3. Fruits 1 medium apple, banana, orange 4. Milk, yogurt 1 cupof milk /yogurt 5. Meat, poultry, fish dry beans, eggs, nuts Approx. 80-100gm of cooked lean meat, poultry, fish, ½ cup of cooked dry beans, 1 egg Meat, Poultry, Fish, Dry Beans, Eggs, & Nuts Group 2-3 SERVINGS Fats, Oils, & Sweets USE SPARINGLY Milk, Yogurt, & Cheese Group 2-3 SERVINGS Vegetable Group 3-5 SERVINGS Pasta Group 6-11 SERVINGS Fruit Group 2-3 SERVINGS 107 lunch and ½ cup dal in the dinner taken together will provide 9½ servings from the bread/cereal group. Vegetarian or non-vegetarian? This is one of the most frequently asked questions, especially by vegetarian sportspersons – Can I compete against non-vegetarians on a vegetarian diet only ? To this question, my answer will be – Yes! Look at these vegetarian sportspersons – 1. Carl Lewis – One of the fastest athletes in the world, in 1991 broke the world record for 100 meters in 9.86 seconds. 2. Martina Navratilova – The first tennis player to win Wimbledon nine times (six being consecutive). 3. Edwin Moses – From 1977 to 1987 achieved 122 victories in the 400 meter hurdles. Won two Olympic gold medals, two world titles, four world records and a streak of 122 consecutive victories. 4. Paavo Nurmi – Great marathon runner, achieved 20 world records with nine Olympic gold medals. In 1924 Olympic Games, he won the 1500 meters and the 5000 meters with just one hour of rest between the two events. The diet of Tarahumara Indians, a tribe of North Central Mexico is mainly vegetarian. They are known for their extraordinary endurance ability. During their popular sport 'Raripuri' the participants run for 150-300 kms, repeat, 150-300 kms! Who is a vegetarian? In fact, vegetarianism has its own different shades. For example, 'Lacto-vegetarians' do not eat meat, fish, fowl and eggs, but they eat dairy products. 'Lacto-ovo-vegetarians' avoid meat, fish and fowls but include 108 dairy products as well as eggs in their diet. 'Vegans' simply avoid all animal products including meat, fish, fowl, eggs, dairy products and even honey. In India, a traditional vegetarian diet falls somewhere in 'Lacto-vegetarian' category. In our analysis, those who rarely consume meat can also be called vegetarians by and large. Advantages of non-vegetarian diet (i) It is rich in protein. (ii) It provides complete protein and has all essential amino acids. Disadvantages of non-vegetarian diet (i) Too much of meat consumption means too much intake of protein. Excess protein intake is fraught with many health risks. Studies have found that diets rich in protein cause excretion of more calcium through urine, thereby increasing the risk of osteoporosis (thinning of bones). (ii) Non-vegetarian diet is high in saturated fats. High intake of saturated fats is associated with major risk factors of cardiovascular disease. (iii) It is high in cholesterol. Again, high cholesterol is associated with major risk factors of cardiovascular disease. (iv) It is low in roughage and therefore promotes constipation. (v) It is low in vitamins. Advice to non-vegetarian (i) Select those animal products which are comparatively low in saturated fats and cholesterol, e.g., chicken is preferable to beef, egg whites to egg yolk. (ii) Consume meat within a reasonable limit to avoid excess intake of protein, saturated fat and cholesterol. (iii) Take adequate carbohydrates. 109 (iv) Include green vegetables and salads in your diet for roughage and essential vitamins. Advantages of vegetarian diet (i) It is high in carbohydrate, the principal source of energy. (ii) A diet based on cereals, vegetables, fruits does not have saturated fats and cholesterol and thereby reduces the major risk factors associated with cardiovascular disease. (iii) It is rich in vitamins and minerals. (iv) It has plenty of roughage facilitating good bowel movement. Disadvantages of vegetarian diet (i) It is generally low in protein. (ii) It does not contain all essential amino-acids. Low protein intake may result into low muscular gain. Advice to vegetarians (i) Combine two or more cereals or vegetable proteins for getting all essential amino acids. For example, combine rice or wheat with soybeans/pulses/legumes/lentils. Actually, this is what traditional Indian diet usually includes. By this method of combination (mutual supplementation), you can compensate individual amino acid deficiency of a vegetable protein. (ii) You can increase protein intake by simply increasing your caloric intake, e.g., take additional cup of moong sprouts or additional cup of milk. (iii) Include low fat dairy products in your diet. 110 II. PROTEINS Importance of proteins (i) Proteins are important for building and repairing of all cells and tissues, including internal organs, muscles, blood cells, brain, bones and skin. (ii) Proteins are components of enzymes and some hormones which regulate our body's activities. (iii) Proteins also provide energy (4k calories/gm) in case of carbohydratedepletion. Carbohydrate-depletion takes place during starvation or prolonged exercise session. However, foods rich in proteins are often expensive and we should not waste them as fuel for energy. Proteins are primarily meant for building and maintenance of the body; carbohydrates and fats are preferred fuel for energy. More protein – more muscles? More protein does not lead to more muscles. In our body, proteins exist in a dynamic state. They are continually broken down and replaced by new proteins. This continued replacement is known as 'protein turnover rate'. Increased physical training, severe illness, hard manual labour etc. increase protein turnover rate. Thus, demand for more proteins arises from within the body. It is not possible to increase the body's protein metabolism artificially and thereby stimulate muscle growth simply by eating more amount of protein. Therefore, you should be careful of the advertisements of high-protein diets claiming to give you a bodybuilder's body without doing any exercises. You might be really pumping your money to the shopkeeper's pocket by eating so much of proteinsupplements! 111 How much proteins do we need? (i) The RDA (Recommended Dietary Allowance) for proteins in adults is .8 gm per kg/body weight per day. If one weighs 70 kg, his daily proteins requirement will be 70 x .8 =56 gm. (ii) Those who are involved in exercise of high intensity and high volume may benefit by taking proteins well above the RDA (1.2-2 gm/ kg body weight/day). Studies show that protein intake beyond 2 gm/kg body weight is not desirable. (iii) Normally, caloric intake from proteins should be 15-20% of the total caloric intake. If one's daily total caloric intake is 3000 Kcalories, 450- 600 Kcalories should come from proteins. Rest of the calories should come from carbohydrates and fats. (iv) Depending upon the nature, intensity and volume of work/ exercise, there can be minor variations in proportion of calories from three major nutrients (i.e., proteins, carbohydrates and fats). For the athletes engaged in strength exercises, 20% of calories may come from proteins, 60% from carbohydrates and 20% from fats. On the other hand, in case of endurance athletes the proportion of carbohydrates may go up to 70%, thereby reducing the caloric percentage from proteins and fats. (v) If there is decrease in total caloric intake for any reason (e.g., in case of someone trying to lose weight by reducing the total caloric intake) he should raise the percentage of caloric intake from proteins above 15% to avoid loss of lean body mass. Lean body mass is the body mass minus fat. The main reason for this is that our major energy requirement should be met from carbohydrates and proteins should be spared for building and maintenance of the body. Proteins are used for energy, only under the extreme conditions, as mentioned earlier. Therefore, if carbohydrate-depletion is a deliberate act and 112 proteins are intended to be used as fuel, total percentage of protein intake will have to be increased above the RDA. What happens to surplus protein? (i) If dietary protein's intake is more than our requirement, it can be utilized by our body for energy or simply converted to fat for future use. (ii) Many of the high-protein diets are high in fat also (e.g., animal foods have large amount of saturated fat and cholesterol). This is a health risk factor. (iii) High-protein diets are often low in fibre. This hampers smooth food movement inside on body and overloads digestive system leading to constipation. (iv) Studies have found that high-protein diet can even cause too much loss of calcium through urine. Those who take high-protein diet should also take high doses of calcium to avoid osteoporosis over a period of time. (v) Excess protein is not good for kidneys. The kidneys would have to process more nitrogenous wastes which are generated during protein metabolism. This overload on kidneys may ultimately lead to kidney disease. (vi) High-protein diets are also more dehydrating. Removal of nitrogenous wastes by kidneys is done through increased fluid excretion causing fluid loss. Dehydration often leads to poor physical and mental performance. Essential and non-essential amino acids Amino acids are building blocks of proteins. There are approximately 22 different amino acids. Ideally, our food should provide all amino acids. The body itself can synthesize some amino acids from carbohydrates (these 113 are called non-essential amino acids). But there are nine amino acids which cannot be synthesized by the body and we have to obtain them from our dietary protein (these are called essential amino acids). Dietary proteins that contain all amino acids (both essential and nonessential amino acids) are known as 'complete proteins'. The complete proteins are generally found in foods of animal sources, i.e., meat, dairy products, eggs, fish, etc. Contrary to this, dietary proteins that do not contain all the amino acids are called 'incomplete proteins'. These are generally of plant origin, e.g., nuts, grains, legumes, seeds, etc. However, vegetarians need not get alarmed by this. By 'mutual supplementation' two or more vegetable proteins can be mixed together to compensate for each other's individual deficiency of all amino acids. For example, soy beans, peas, beans, lentils, legumes can be mixed with rice, wheat, corn etc. This way vegetarian proteins can be as good (and as complete) as non-vegetarian proteins. III. CARBOHYDRATES Introduction The main function of carbohydrates is to supply energy. Though carbohydrates provide approximately equal amount of energy as proteins (4Kcalories/gm), they are far more efficient fuel than proteins. Dietary carbohydrates are of two types – simple and complex. Simple carbohydrates are made up of one or two sugar molecules (e.g., honey, jelly, soft drinks, etc.). Complex carbohydrates contain many sugar molecules linked together. (e.g., whole grains, potatoes, vegetables and fruits, etc.). How much carbohydrates should we take? (i) As per the RDA, (Recommended Dietary Allowance) our daily carbohydrates intake should be within range of 6-11 gm/kg of body 114 weight. If a person weighs 70 kg, he should take 420-770gms of carbohydrates depending upon his daily caloric requirement. A 70-kg marathoner will require more caloric intake (and, thereby, proportionately more carbohydrates) than a 70-kg sedentary clerk. (ii) 55-60% of our total dietary calories should come from carbohydrates. If a person's daily caloric intake is 3000 calories, 1650-1800 calories should come from carbohydrates. (iii) Carbohydrates are a preferred metabolic fuel. They spare proteins for muscle building and maintenance of body. If our intake of Carbohydrates is less than the RDA, our body may tend to utilize proteins for energy and consequently muscle building may suffer. (iv) Low carbohydrate diet will build up low glycogen stores in the muscles. Thus, chronically deplete muscle glycogen stores may lead a person to reduced performance. Those on 'crash diet' should note this. Digestion of carbohydrates Digestion of carbohydrates starts in mouth. While chewing of food (mastication) we produce saliva. Salivary enzyme amylase breaks down the starch(which is tasteless) of carbohydrate to maltose which is sweet. This is why food tastes sweet if properly chewed. During digestion carbohydrates are broken down into glucose and circulated in blood to be used for energy. If our body does not use glucose immediately for energy, surplus glucose is converted into glycogen and stored in muscles and liver for future use. Approximately, 2/3 glycogen is stored in muscles and 1/3 in liver. Since total glucose storage capacity of muscles and liver is limited, the surplus amount of glycogen is converted and stored as fat. This is why overeating causes more fat deposit in body. 115 Chewing our food well helps better digestion and optimal utilization of food intake. Yoga teachers recommend to 'drink the food' (chew the food so long that it becomes liquid in your mouth, then swallow it) for its best utilization. Chewing well also discourages overeating. (The task itself is so boring that naturally you will not have much patience to take huge dose of food !) Complex vs simple carbohydrates Complex carbohydrates are preferable to simple carbohydrates for these reasons – (i) Complex carbohydrates contain fibre, water, vitamins and other nutrients. Simple carbohydrates on the other hand, have hardly any other nutrients. (ii) The presence of fibres in whole-grain food makes them more satisfying. Foods rich in fibre prevent constipation. (iii) High-fibre foods, also take more calories for their digestion. This has an important implication for weight control. One can eat high-fibre foods to his satisfaction and still may not gain much weight! (iv) Complex carbohydrates encourage better glycogen storage than simple sugars. Carbohydrates loading (carbo-loading) Carbo-loading is a practice prevalent among endurance athletes. This technique is used to enhance muscle glycogen store of the athlete prior to the race. Firstly, the athlete eats low-carbohydrates diet for 3 days and simultaneously has prolonged exercise sessions of high-intensity to deplete his body of the carbohydrates to a great extent. This is followed by 3 days of rest or very low-intensity exercise and simultaneously a highcarbohydrates diet. During these 3 days, a 'carbo-starved' body tends to store more muscle glycogen than its normal level (super-compensation 116 effect). This increased level of glycogen store helps the athlete to perform for a longer time. 'Hitting the wall' is an experience that occurs to runners during long distance runs (e.g., during marathon) when marathoner's body is so depleted of carbohydrates that he seems to 'hit the wall' and has hardly any energy left in him to carry forward. Carbo-loading pushes the 'wall' further towards the finishing line. (If earlier you hit the wall at 30th km, now you may experience it, may be, at 40th km.) However, this technique does not suit everyone. Sometimes carbo-loading in its carbo-depletion stage causes undesirable side effects, e.g., physical and mental fatigue, depression and irritability. Never try this at the time of race unless you have done so during your training. Tips to make the most out of carbohydrates: (i) Carbohydrates are best absorbed if taken immediately after the exercise. Why? A prolonged, intense exercise causes carbohydratesdepletion in our body. The muscle glycogen level requires to be restored soon after the exercise. If carbohydrates are not ingested within half an hour or so, our body turns to utilize its proteins for energy requirement. As mentioned earlier, proteins are primarily meant for body building and not for supplying energy. If they are diverted to be used as fuel, muscle building will take a back seat. (ii) What's the best type of carbohydrates for instant refuelling after exercise? A natural choice will be those carbohydrates that figure high on glycemic index. (Glycemic index is a scale that describes how fast a food is converted to glucose in the blood). However, in some cases, taking too much of high glycemic carbohydrates may elevate blood-sugar level. This may stimulate sudden spurt of insulin which may cause abnormal fall in the blood-sugar level (hypoglycemia). Due to temporary hypoglycemia, one may feel weak or dizzy. Therefore, it 117 is advised to have a wise combination of both high and low glycemic foods. Most fruits and vegetables, whole grain breads, milk, dals are low glycemic Index foods. Cornflakes, potatoes, watermelon, white bread, sugar, honey are high foods. Major sources of carbohydrates are rice, wheat, jowar, ragi, potato, tapioca, banana, honey, fruits. IV. FATS Introduction Fats are not as bad as most of us are made to believe. On the contrary, they are useful in many ways - (i) They help in absorption of fat- soluble vitamins, i.e., vitamin A, vitamin D, vitamin E and vitamin K. Vitamin A is required for growth and repair of tissues, maintenance of proper vision, resistance to infection; Vitamin D is required for bones and teeth; Vitamin E helps in the muscle tissue/repair process; Vitamin K is required in the process of blood clotting, protein formation and also for healthy bones. (ii) Fats provide energy. (iii) Let's be honest about it, fats make our food tasty. (iv) Essential fats (those fats which our body cannot make; therefore, we have to get them from food) are required for our normal growth, healthy arteries and nerves, for smooth skin and healthy joints. They also help in cholesterol metabolism. Corn, soybean, safflower oils are very high in essential fats. Nuts, seeds are also very important source of essential fats. 118 (v) Studies have shown that Omega-3 fatty acids (found mainly in fish as well as in green leafy vegetables, nuts) are helpful for the patients of heart disease and high blood pressure. They help to make high density lipoprotein (HDL) and regulate production of low density lipoprotein (LDL). (vi) Fats regulate sex hormones. (vii) Fats are necessary for healthy cells. How much fat is enough? (i) American Heart Association (AHA) recommends that in our daily diet not more than 30% of total calories should come from fat. However, in case of bodybuilders, athletes, who have to carry more muscle mass than fat in their body composition for peak performance, fat may come form 15-20% of their total calories. For a normal person 20% dietary fat is enough. (ii) Saturated fats should contribute not more than 30% of the total calories from fats. (iii) However, by reducing fat intake less than 15-30%of total dietary calories you risk trouble in absorption of fat-soluble vitamins (vitamins A, D, E, K). Saturated, unsaturated and trans fats The classification of fats is based on the saturation of their chemical bonds by hydrogen. In saturated fatty acids most of the chemical bonds are occupied by hydrogen. Unsaturated fats have fewer of these bonds occupied by hydrogen. Animal fats are available in meat, egg, milk and milk products. These fats are predominantly saturated and associated with heart disease. Therefore, their consumption should be limited. Vegetable fats are predominantly unsaturated. Unsaturated fats are mostly liquid at room 119 temperature (e.g., vegetable oils). Saturated fats are mostly solid at room temperature. However, coconut oil is an exception, which is saturated but exists as a liquid at room temperature. Trans fats are produced when liquid fat is made solid by a process called hydrogenation. Trans fats act like saturated fats and can pose the same health risks. Many of the processed foods like potato chips, samosa, bakery items (cakes, muffins, cookies, etc.), french fries contain trans fats. Why excess dietary fat is not good for you: When we count the fat intake in our diet, we should not overlook the hidden fat. For example, while munching deep fried peanuts we should not forget that in addition to the oil used for cooking, the peanuts themselves contain huge amount of fats. These are some inherent health risks involved with high-fat diet − (i) There is a relationship between dietary fat (especially saturated fat), blood cholesterol level and risk of heart disease. The risk of colon cancer is also associated with high-fat diet. (ii) Unsaturated fats contribute to production of free radicals which are associated with aging and certain degenerative diseases. (iii) Fat has less thermic effect. This means that fewer calories are required to convert dietary fat into body fat. This contributes to weight gain. (iv) Fat is a high-energy source. (Protein/carbohydrates?4 kcalories/gm; fat?9 kcalories/gm). It satisfies appetite very readily and is stored in body very easily. This may discourage one to take balanced food if his hunger is already satisfied. Cholesterol Cholesterol is a waxy, light-coloured substance. It comes in two different forms- cholesterol in food and cholesterol in blood. Our dietary cholesterol intake should not exceed 300mg/day. Food cholesterol is 120 mainly found in foods of animal origin (meat, dairy products). Plant foods do not contain any cholesterol. Foods like liver, eggs, beef, pork, chicken, milk are high in cholesterol. Our liver manufactures blood cholesterol from saturated fats. This means that the more saturated fat we take the more cholesterol our liver will make. The excess circulation of cholesterol in blood can accumulate on the inner walls of the arteries (called plaque) leading to heart disease. Cholesterol may be present in blood as a constituent of Low Density Lipoprotein (LDL) or of High Density Lipoprotein (HDL). LDL and HDL affect heart disease risk differently. LDL is known as bad cholesterol. It is responsible for depositing cholesterol on the artery walls. HDL is good cholesterol. It contains smaller amount of cholesterol. Its job is to remove cholesterol from the cells in the artery walls and transport it back to the liver for reprocessing . V. VITAMINS AND MINERALS Introduction Vitamins and minerals are referred to as micronutrients. Unlike macronutrients (i.e., proteins, carbohydrates and fats) they do not directly supply energy. But they help in the metabolism of macronutrients. Vitamins Vitamins are organic substances. They cannot be synthesized by our body. Therefore, they are to be obtained from our diet. Vitamins are classified according to their solubility in fat or water. There are four fat-soluble vitamins – vitamins A, D, E and K. They are absorbed with dietary fats and can be stored to some extent in our body. Water-soluble vitamins are – vitamin C, B1 , B2 , B6 , B12, niacin, folic acid etc. Unlike fat soluble vitamins, these vitamins are not normally stored 121 in the body. Therefore, we have to take them daily. Symptoms of watersoluble vitamins deficiency may be apparent in 6-7 days. How much vitamins do we require? One of the most frequently asked questions is whether one requires vitamins supplements. The answer is – generally, there is no cause of worry about vitamins deficiency if one is on a nutritionally balanced diet. This applies to athletes also. However, in case of very intense/high-volume exercise, one may require to take vitamin/mineral supplementation. Studies have shown that heavy exercise may reduce vitamin/mineral status in the body. This generally happens in case of vitamin C and riboflavin (B2). Stressful situations may increase the need for vitamins and minerals too. But one should remember that generally the increased requirement for vitamins and minerals can be met by proportionately increasing total amount of diet. Sometimes, high doses of vitamins may produce a temporary feeling of improved performance. But remember that vitamins taken in abnormally high doses, are no longer working as vitamins only; possibly they are acting like performance-enhancing drugs. 122 Functions of major vitamins and their food sources are given in the table below – Vitamins Functions Best Food Sources Vitamin A Normal vision, growth and repair of body tissues Liver, egg yolk, whole milk, butter, carrot, ghee, papaya, green leafy vegetables. Vitamin D Helps in absorption of calcium and building of bone mass. Fish, milk, egg yolks, butter and sunlight. Vitamin E Helps in repairs of exercise- induced tissue damage Nuts, seeds, wheat germ, polyunsaturated vegetable oils, fish liver oils, peanut butter Vitamin K For normal blood clotting, bone formation Vegetables, milk. Vitamin C Helps iron absorption, protects against infections. Amla, Citrus fruits and green leafy vegetables, lemon juice, potatoes. Vitamin BComplex Metabolism of carbohydrates, proteins, fats, healthy nervous system, normal growth. Rice, wheat, animal foods, nuts, peanuts, soybean, leafy vegetables, fruits, beans. Minerals Minerals are inorganic elements constituting approximately 3-4% of our body weight. These are generally divided into two categories – (i) Trace elements – these minerals are present in very small quantities, i.e., less than .01% of body weight; (ii) Macrominerals – they are more then .01% of body weight. Both are equally important for our body and their deficiency may have major health implications. The macrominerals include sodium, calcium, phosphorus, magnesium, potassium, sulphur. Important trace 123 elements are iron, zinc, selenium, iodine. We will discuss about some important minerals. Sodium Sodium maintains normal water balance within our body, affects blood pressure, maintains acid-base balance and muscular contraction. The major sources of sodium are common salt (Sodium Chloride) and MSG (Monosodium Glutamate). One tea spoon of salt (approx. 5 gm) has approximately 2000-2200 milligram of sodium. Sodium is naturally found in majority of the foods. The recommended sodium intake is around 500-2400 mg a day (i.e. not more than approximately 1¼ tea spoon). Most of us eat more salt and thus take more sodium than we actually need. This will be evident when we notice the 'hidden salt' in our foods – both natural as well as processed. Junk foods are bad due to their high salt contents also. Excess sodium intake can cause water retention in our body which may result into undesirable weight gain. Don't be surprised if one fine morning your weighing machine suddenly shows a weight gain of 200-400 gm. In all probability, the culprit may be just the small salty pickle you ate previous night! Secondly, high salt intake may increase the risk of high blood pressure. Thirdly, too much of salt is bad for our kidneys. There are two myths associated with salt – (i) one requires more salt while doing vigorous and prolonged exercise, and (ii) cramps can be avoided (especially during distance running), if salt intake is increased. The fact is that actual loss of salt through sweat is not very significant. If we look at our daily amount of salt intake, we will find that our daily intake of salt is enough for running a marathon per day! Secondly, the studies have yet to find any substantive relationship between muscle cramps and salt deficiency. 124 Calcium Calcium and Phosphorous are major constituents of our bones and teeth. Every day some amount of calcium from the bones circulates in the blood. This removed amount of bone calcium is quickly replaced by calcium from our diet. If the dietary calcium is not adequate, the lost bone calcium cannot be fully replaced. Calcium deficiency may thus lead to inadequate bone calcification and subsequently to osteoporosis. Dairy products are major sources of calcium. Therefore, those who avoid intake of dairy products in their diet (for fear of weight gain) are at a greater risk. Increasing calcium content of diet may be useful to prevent osteoporosis. Physical exercise, particularly weight training, may also help prevent and reverse osteoporosis. Weight training increases the density of bones by stressing them. Therefore, the best way to prevent osteoporosis will be to combine both exercise and diet. There is a word of caution for those who are engaged in long-distance running. Their diet may not be adequate enough to provide sufficient calcium for replacement of lost bone calcium. In their cases, prolonged exercise may lead to bone-thinning instead of bone-strengthening. Such athletes should seek medical advice to increase their calcium intake accordingly. Iron Iron deficiency is found to be common among athletes, especially, those involved in prolonged physical activities (e.g., long-distance running). This deficiency may be due to inadequate absorption of dietary iron, losses from gastrointestinal tract, or excessive sweating. The RDA for iron is 10 mg/day for men and 15 mg/per day for women. Women require more iron than men because of iron losses during their menstruation. 125 Since iron is necessary for carrying oxygen to muscles, iron deficiency may lead to less oxygen supply to muscles. This deficiency may result into extreme fatigue, loss of strength and endurance, and prolonged recovery periods after an exercise. Iron is found in two forms. Heme iron (in animal foods, e. g., meat, liver, poultry, fish) is readily absorbed iron. Non-heme iron (in vegetables) is less absorbed. Your body is not able to absorb all iron present in the vegetables. However, there are certain food items that help in more absorption of non-heme iron, e. g., foods rich in Vitamin C. Add some fruit or a glass of fruit juice, or salad to your diet, or simply sprinkle some lemon juice for better absorption of iron from vegetables. Coffee and tea tend to inhibit the absorption of iron. Hence, these beverages should be taken 1-2 hrs. after the meal. On the other hand, excess iron intake has its own harmful implications. It tends to cause indigestion and constipation. In its extreme form excess iron intake may lead to hemochromatoris, in which the body stores excess iron in heart and liver tissue. 126 Functions of important minerals and their food sources are given in the following table – Mineral Function Best Food Sources A. Major Minerals Calcium Healthy bones, teeth, muscle contraction. Dairy products, green leafy vegetables, Ragi. Phosphorous Strong bones and teeth. Animal foods, whole grains, nuts. Magnesium Metabolism of carbohydrates and proteins. Whole grains, nuts, green vegetables. Potassium Maintenance of normal fluid balance of cells, muscle contraction. Potatoes, vegetables, fruits, banana. Sodium Maintenance of normal fluid balance of cells, Nerve and muscle function. In almost all foods B. Trace Iron Red blood cell formation, oxygen transport to cells. Green leafy vegetable, liver, meats, nuts, beans. Iodine Regulation of growth, development, energy metabolism. Iodized salt. VI. WATER Importance of water By weight, water constitutes approximately 45-60% of human body. Water provides a medium for biochemical reactions as well as transport and exchange of nutrients, metabolic by-products, gases and heat. Therefore, any small change in water content in our body may cause changes in 127 biochemical reaction dependent on water. Acute water loss, i.e., dehydration may bring many health complications. Sufficient water intake is necessary for healthy kidneys. Inadequate water intake increases concentration of urine and thus contributes to stones formation as well as growth of germs infections. The best way to avoid these complications is to keep urine sufficiently dilute by drinking sufficient water throughout the day. One body loses water through perspiration and respiration. Depending upon intensity and duration of exercise or outside temperature, a person may lose between 1-3 litres of water per hour (i.e., approximately 1-3 kg of body weight). Any intense exercise beyond one hour will thus interfere with cooling function of the body and will affect a person's performance. A marathon runner may lose even upto 4.5 litres of water during 2½-3 hrs. of race. This loss cannot be compensated during the race and there will be a huge deficit of water intake. It is, therefore, important to hydrate one's body before, during and after any prolonged exercise. Guidelines for adequate hydration: (i) Don't wait for thirst. The feeling of thirst lags behind your body's need for water. Therefore, without waiting for thirst, drink sufficient amount of water in a day. The colour of your urine is a good indicator of your body's hydration. It should always be clear or pale; if it is yellowish, it may be indicative of under-hydration. (ii) Cold water (4-5 0C) is absorbed faster in your system. However, during cold day warm water will make you more comfortable. (iii) On higher altitudes, where it is dry, drink more water. (iv) Avoid coffee, tea, cola, alcohol. These are diuretics (diuretics cause the body to eliminate water and thus dehydrate it). It is a good idea to drink a glass of water before drinking tea or coffee. 128 (v) During an exercise of a longer duration (beyond 1 hour), drink (100-150 ml) every 15-20 minutes. But never 'over drink'. (vi) Sugar-and-electrolyte solutions can be taken during prolonged exercise, but they should be sufficiently diluted. It should be a hypotonic solution with a lower osmotic pressure than that of body's fluids. If the solution is too concentrated, it will not be absorbed by the body and can lead to gastric distress. Taking glucose in dry powder form is not a good practice. Hyponatremia (water intoxication) It is good to hydrate oneself at regular intervals during an exercise of long duration. But too much of water intake has its own hazards. Over drinking may lead to hyponatremia (loss of sodium). This happens as too much of water ingestion dilutes sodium contents in blood. Acute sodiumdeficiency may result into heat exhaustion and cardiovascular collapse. Summary of the chapter – Nothing is as confusing as the subject of nutrition. Don't get confused. Be practical. Eat whatever you have been eating and enjoying so far. Just keep following points in your mind regarding your diet – (i) Proportion of daily calories should approximately follow this formula – 60% from carbohydrates, 20% from protein and 20% from fats. (ii) Avoid processed, tinned food (which are high in sugar, salts and low in fibres). Prefer natural, seasonal, fresh, fibrous food. (iii) Follow Food Guide Pyramid. (iv) Reduce your salt intake. Excess salt adds to high blood pressure. It also adds to overall body weight by retaining more water in body. (v) Include nuts in your diet. 129 (vi) Eat sprouts of Bengal gram, moong, soybeans,etc. They are filled with enzymes, protein, complex carbohydrates, fibre, vitamin and minerals. Sprouts also contain antioxidants and protect us from the ongoing effects of aging. (vii) Cut down on sugar. (viii) Cut down on saturated fats. Prefer low fat diet. (ix) Avoid overeating. Eat 4-5 small meals instead throughout the day. (x) Be happy while eating your food.

The secret to why nutrition is essential for people is in the word itself – nutrition comes from nutrients. Nutrients are the good things that we get through food which we need to nourish and nurture ourselves, and to be happy and healthy people.

In scientific terms, nutrition is the supply of food that we need as an organism to feed our cells and keep them alive. We can get nutrients from products such as vitamin supplements, however when we talk about nutrition we mostly mean the nutrients we get from food.

Nutrition means getting the food and nourishment that you need for health and growth.

Without nutrition, we grow weak, sick and at the very worst can even die. We miss developmental milestones and can't put our bodies through the daily mental and physical tasks that we need them to. We aren't able to grow and may also be unable to reproduce.

Nutrients are the fuel we need to enable the body to break down food and then put this to use in the body to repair and build cells and tissue, which is basically our metabolism.

The healthy human body needs seven different kinds of nutrients to thrive; proteins, carbohydrates, fats, vitamins, minerals, fibre and water. Macronutrients are the ones we need lots of, while with micronutrients (the vitamins and minerals) we can get by with a bit less.

Many of them fuel energy, while others have other important roles like digestion and hydration.

Micronutrients: little, but very important

Vitamins are the most commonly known micronutrients, which are essential organic compounds that the body needs to function but which it can't create on its own. There are thirteen different vitamins people need including A, D, E, K, eight different B vitamins, and C.

Other micronutrients are the minerals, which we don't need in as large a quantity as the other nutrients listed, but there is a wide range of minerals that we should be getting, which can make it difficult to get them all.

The minerals we need include magnesium, iron, zinc, potassium, calcium, chloride, sodium, manganese, copper, and several more. There are 16 different minerals that we need to thrive.

What is a nutritional imbalance?

A nutritional imbalance happens when you are not getting the right amounts of all of the nutrients you need. You can have too much of something, but it is generally more serious to have too little of a nutrient.

To help maintain your body and keep it strong you need to have a balanced diet as well as a nutritional one.

Different nutrients have very different jobs in the body and show up as different kinds of deficiency when they are lacking.

If you are missing all of the nutrients in general, such as being completely deprived of food and water then you can become malnourished.

You can become deficient in certain nutrients for a number of reasons:

Not consuming enough of them

Your body has difficulty processing one or more

Disease

Medications can deplete them

Stress

Your digestive system isn't working properly

You have an allergy or sensitivity to certain nutrients

Nutritional imbalances or deficiencies are usually very easily tested for, and in most cases can also be easily remedied.

Easy ways to improve your nutrition

The best way to get the nutrition you need is through your diet. The body usually processes food better than supplements, so this is the most effective and efficient way to get what you need.

But if diet can't do it because you can't get the food you need or your body won't tolerate it, then supplements are available to, well, supplement your diet and nutrition needs.

Pay attention to your body and any changes

Your body's needs will change over time. Babies and children need different nutrients and quantities to adults, men need different amounts to women, and then pregnant or menopausal women need different again.

If you have a sensitivity to any food, which can also develop later in life, your needs will change again. You may have processed certain foods wonderfully when you were younger but develop problems with them with age, including carbohydrates and other sugars.

Pay attention to what your body needs and how you feel. If you are lacking in energy or having trouble with your digestion, this can be an early sign that something might be out of balance.

Get a check-up

If anything seems out of balance, you should talk to your doctor about tests for nutritional imbalances; most of these can be done with simple blood tests.

Even if nothing feels wrong you should still have a regular check-up with your doctor to keep an eye on your changing and ageing body.

Eat a regular, balanced and nutritious diet

People need to consume around 2000 calories a day, usually across 3 to 6 meals. Eating a healthy diet means not going over that amount too often, trying not to skip meals, because we tend to overcompensate for it later, and to get our daily calorie allowance from the right foods.

Around half of what we eat should be fruit and vegetables in a wide range of colours – the broader the rainbow the better. Then around a quarter of our intake should come from proteins like meat, chicken, fish, legumes, dairy and nuts, and around a quarter from carbohydrates like wholegrains and starchy vegetables.

We should eat very little fat or sugar that has been added to food and instead get both our fats and energy intake from the sources we listed above. Healthy fats come from proteins and things like avocados and olive oil, while healthy sugars come from fruit and dairy.

Look into supplements to help

For many people, adding a daily supplement to help their nutrient intake along is an excellent idea. If you aren't able to get nutrients from their most natural source then supplements are a great and easy option.

Particularly for people with high vitamin needs like pregnant women or those recovering from serious illness, it would be virtually impossible to get what you need from food alone.

Tips to Keep the Weight Off

Meeting your goal weight is just the first step in making healthy lifestyle adjustments. You have a better chance of keeping the weight off if you incorporate things like exercise goals, eating whole foods, and spending less time in front of television and computer screens.

What are some tips to keep a healthy weight?

Now that you've reached your goal weight, you will need to continue to make healthy lifestyle changes so you don't regain the weight you've lost. The National Weight Control Registry (NWCR) provides success stories of more than 10,000 people who have lost weight and kept it off. If you want to avoid regaining weight, keep a positive attitude and use the guidelines below.

Exercise often: Studies prove that people with high activity levels are more likely to maintain their weight loss than others who are not as active. Set exercise goals, aiming to build up to a minimum of 200-300 minutes of exercise per week (ACSM guidelines).

Eat a healthy breakfast daily. Seventy-eight percent of participants in the NWCR eat breakfast every day.

Stay hydrated. Drink plenty of water or other no-calorie unsweetened beverages. Avoid sugar-sweetened beverages.

Eat whole foods. Focus on a healthy eating pattern of whole, unprocessed foods that is rich in produce and fiber, contains lean protein sources, and is lower in fat.

Eat responsibly and mindfully. Pay attention to portion sizes and avoid overeating. Look at the nutrition facts on food labels listed on packages, including the serving size. Using smaller plates and bowls may help you choose smaller portions at meals. Prioritize meal time. Eat slowly, with focus on your meal. Listen to your body 's physical cues to stop eating before you feel overly full. On special occasions, choose your foods as wisely as you would on any other day.

Plan your meals ahead of time. By planning meals in advance, you can make healthier choices that are not influenced by physical hunger. Plan home-cooked meals, reserving restaurant dining for special occasions. Packing low-calorie snacks like fresh fruits, vegetables and whole grains can help keep hunger controlled throughout the day.

Get cookbooks. Need extra ideas for meals? Try some different recipes to avoid getting bored with your healthier diet choices. Great recipes can be found in cookbooks at the public library, bookstores or on the Internet.

Decrease screen time. More time in front of the television or computer means less time on your feet using calories. Sixty-two percent of NWCR participants watch less than 10 hours of TV per week. Choose enjoyable activities that keep you on your feet and moving during leisure time. This movement is important in addition to exercise time.

Monitor yourself. If you don't hold yourself accountable, who will? Weigh yourself weekly, or take self measurements regularly; 75% of participants in the NWCR weigh themselves at least once a week. If you find yourself going back to old habits, try to keep a record of food and exercise for a few weeks until you get back on track.

Join a weight management program. The longer and more often you are engaged, the better long-term success.

Build a support group. Find a friend or family member who can listen and relate to what you are going through. Invite them to join you and make the changes together.

Keep a positive attitude. Believe in yourself! Keep in mind that some days will be better than others. When you have a day of overeating, learn to pick yourself up and move on. Each new day is a fresh start for healthy eating.

Think for the long term. A diet is only a short-term method or tool to lose weight. In order to continue to keep the weight off, long-term changes need to be made. Rethink your old ways of eating and identify habits that caused you to gain weight. Consider what, when, why, where, and how you eat. Make any changes necessary for a more healthful eating lifestyle. For example, did you previously overeat at night while watching television in the family room? If so, make a change to stop eating in the family room or in front of the television. Instead, eat only in the kitchen at the table.

Make gradual turns. Plan one change at a time that can be incorporated into your new lifestyle. Once you have mastered it, plan another change. Studies prove that the longer people can maintain their new weight, the easier it becomes. Take one step at a time, and you will be headed for success.

Skip the absolutes. Stay away from words like "never," "always" or "must." Be realistic with yourself and allow indulgences on occasion. You should be able to have your favorite treats without feeling guilty. Smaller portions of higher calorie foods can be worked into your new eating style. Thoroughly enjoy each bite instead of fixating on what you can't have.

Make an appointment with a registered dietitian (RD). If you need expert advice for nutrition information, don't hesitate to make an appointment with a registered dietitian. He or she can provide helpful tips and point you in the right direction for a healthy lifestyle change.

Continue your healthy eating habits. You have done a great job to get to where you are now. Keep updating your goals as new situations arise.

As you grow older, if you continue eating the same types and amounts of food but do not become more active, you will probably gain weight. That's because your metabolism (how your body gets energy from food) can slow with age, and your body composition (amount of fat and muscle) may be different from when you were younger.

The energy your body gets from the nutrients in the food you eat is measured as calories. As a rule of thumb, the more calories you eat, the more active you have to be to maintain your weight. Likewise, the reverse is also true—the more active you are, the more calories you need. As you age, your body might need less food for energy, but it still needs the same amount of nutrients.

Many things can affect your weight, including genetics, age, gender, lifestyle, family habits and culture, sleep, and even where you live and work. Some of these factors can make it hard to lose weight or keep weight off.

But being active and choosing healthy foods has health benefits for everyone—no matter your age or weight. It's important to choose nutrient-dense foods and be active at least 150 minutes per week. As a rule of thumb:

To keep your weight the same, you need to burn the same number of calories as you eat and drink.

To lose weight, burn more calories than you eat and drink.

To gain weight, burn fewer calories than you eat and drink.

Read and Share this infographic and help spread the word about healthy diet and exercise.

Tips for Maintaining a Healthy Weight

Limit portion size to control calorie intake.

Add healthy snacks during the day if you want to gain weight.

Be as physically active as you can be.

Talk to your doctor about your weight if you think that you weigh too much or too little.

What Should I Eat to Maintain a Healthy Weight?

Choose foods that have a lot of nutrients but not a lot of calories. NIA has information to help you make healthy food choices and shop for food that's good for you.

How Much Physical Activity Do I Need?

Aim for at least 150 minutes of moderate-intensity aerobic activity each week. You don't have to do that all at once—break it up over the whole week, however you like. If you can't do this much activity right away, try to be as physically active as you can. Doing something is better than doing nothing at all.

The benefits of exercise aren't just about weight. Regular exercise can make it easier for you to do daily activities, participate in outings, drive, keep up with grandchildren, avoid falls, and stay independent.

Tip: Physical Activity

Most older people can be moderately active. But, you might want to talk to your doctor if you aren't used to energetic activity and you want to start a vigorous exercise program or significantly increase your physical activity. You should also check with your doctor if you have health concerns like the following:

Dizziness

Shortness of breath

Chest pain or pressure

An irregular heartbeat

Blood clots

Joint swelling

A hernia

Recent hip or back surgery

Your doctor might have some safety tips or suggest certain types of exercise for you.

You don't have to spend a lot of money joining a gym or hiring a personal trainer. Think about the kinds of physical activities that you enjoy—for example, walking, running, bicycling, gardening, housecleaning, swimming, or dancing. Try to make time to do what you enjoy on most days of the week. And then increase how long you do it, or add another fun activity.

Five Strategies for Healthy Weight Management

The new year is a popular time to set a weight management goal. Eating better, exercising more, and losing weight are consistently among the top resolutions made in January and beyond. However, while many individuals begin with the best intentions, few of them actually stick to a resolution for the entire year.

If you're making one, then to make sure you hit your healthy weight goal this year, we have outlined five strategies to help you on your weight management journey.

Five Ways to Manage Weight

1. Eat more filling foods

Not all foods fill you up equally. For example, a bowl of oatmeal in the morning is more filling than a bowl of sugar-packed cereal. What you eat can determine how full you feel and can help avoid hunger pangs and temptation between meals. Foods that enable you to feel full for a longer period are generally high in protein, fiber, and water content. Some examples of these types of foods are:

Avocados

Lentils

Whole grains

Black beans

Bananas

Brussels sprouts

2. Plan meals in advance

Another way to cut back on calories is to plan your meals in advance. It is easier to stick to a healthy diet when you pre-plan the portions of each meal, and it helps to avoid spontaneous temptations while preparing the meal.

Meal planning can seem daunting at first, but it can be approached in three simple steps.

Plan your meals on Friday. Look at the following week's schedule and decide on the recipes you want to make.

Shop for your meals on Saturday. Once you have the recipes in mind, create your list and shop for the ingredients.

Prep your meals on Sunday for the week ahead.

3. Find physical activities you enjoy

The more you exercise the better. But it's hard to commit to exercise if you aren't having fun. If lifting weights or early morning running isn't your thing, then don't sweat it. Find something you do enjoy instead. To find a more enjoyable fitness habit, ask yourself the following:

Do you prefer working out alone or in a group?

Where do you prefer to work out? At home or in a gym? Inside or outdoors?

What's most convenient for you? The fewer obstacles you have, the easier it is to commit to exercising.

4. Manage your stress

An often-overlooked aspect of weight management is stress management. Stress results in multiple unhealthy behaviors and moods – such as overeating (especially junk food), skipping meals entirely, and messing with sleep schedules – all of which have adverse effects when it comes to weight management.

Before starting any weight management routine, measure your stress levels. Thorne's At-Home Stress Test measures the two primary biomarkers of stress – cortisol and DHEA – which will enable you to know if you are managing your stress effectively or if you need to do more.

5. Supplement your weight management strategies

Everyone's weight management goals are different. Some individuals want better health and increased energy. Others want to maintain a healthy lifestyle and avoid illness.

No matter what your goals are, Thorne's Weight Management Bundle can help because, along with diet and regular exercise, nutritional supplementation is an important factor in supporting the body's metabolism.*

The secret to reaching your goal isn't some crazy diet. The real magic lies in simple math.

The key to shedding pounds isn't jumping into whatever fad diet is popular at the moment. No, the smartest game plan for those in the know doesn't involve eating a lot of one kind of food (we're looking at you, grapefruit diet) or living off of only liquids for days at a time (seriously, why would you want to do that?). It's actually reaching for a calculator and using some basic math to help subtract all that unwanted fat.

Getting to a body weight you feel comfortable with means reminding yourself how many calories your body actually needs each day to function at its best. Once you know that number, losing weight and feeling great is as easy as trimming back a reasonable number of calories while burning off a few more with exercise. Grab your pencils:

Step 1:

Find out how many calories your body needs each day to maintain your current weight. Just take your current weight and multiply it by 13 (if you don't exercise at all), 15 (if you exercise a few times weekly) or 18 (if you exercise five days or more a week). The number you'll be left with is a rough idea of how many calories you're most likely eating right now.

For example, if you weigh 165 pounds and exercise three days a week, then you would multiply 165 by 15 for a total of 2,475. That means your daily calorie intake—and how you will stay stuck at your current weight—is about 2,475 calories.

Step 2:

Reduce your daily calorie intake by between 500 to 1,000 calories. You can create this calorie deficit one of three ways:

1. You can eat 500 to 1,000 fewer calories each day.

2. You can burn off 500 to 1,000 calories each day through exercise.

3. You can combine a little of both, eating 250 to 500 fewer calories while burning 250 to 500 calories each day, for example.

Why not more? Most experts agree that losing between 1 and 2 pounds weekly is a safer, sounder approach to weight loss. Since 1 pound of fat equals approximately 3,500 calories, by reducing your caloric intake by 3,500 to 7,000 calories each week, you'll safely lose about 1 to 2 pounds each week.

Keep in mind: Your daily calorie intake—the calories you eat—should never dip below 1,200 (for women) or 1,800 (for men). Eating any less than that can rob your body of the nutrients it needs to be healthy. To be sure you're reaching your ideal calorie intake, consider using a free tracking tool, like MyFitnessPal. Through the website or app, you can easily record exactly what you eat each day. And because you can search and add specific foods and serving sizes (a cup of low-fat Greek yogurt, for example) all the work of counting is done for you, making tracking super simple.

Step 3:

Remember that anything can be exercise. If you hate running or weight training, there are plenty of other options that can help melt away body fat. Here are just a few ways to burn 100 calories (based on a 150-pound person).

• Swimming or taking a cardio dance class for 15 minutes (moderate intensity)

• Walking (at a pace of 3.5 miles per hour), shooting hoops, mowing the lawn, or painting a room for 20 minutes

• Casual biking or playing with your children for 23 minutes

Step 4:

Repeat step 1 every week to discover your new daily calorie intake. That may sound obvious, but a lot of people tend to follow the same diet plan for months—even years—then wonder why they never seem to lose weight. They forget that after their body becomes 1 or 2 pounds lighter, it doesn't need as many calories to sustain that new weight. But by using the formula every week, you'll always know exactly how much you should be eating to reach your goal and never hit .

Weight cycling is losing weight and regaining it over and over. It's called "yo-yo" dieting when it happens because of dieting.

Weight cycles can be big (50 pounds or more) or small (5-10 pounds).

Is it bad for you? That's not clear. Staying overweight isn't healthy, so ask your doctor what your goal weight should be, what you should do to reach that weight, and what it takes to stay at that weight.

Your doctor may not have all the answers, so ask them for a referral to a dietitian to help you find ways to eat better and lose extra weight. Working with a personal trainer will help you get on track with exercise, which is especially important in keeping the pounds off once you reach your goal weight.

You can break the cycle of losing and regaining weight. Researchers showed that by following 439 overweight women for a year. The women who had a history of moderate or big weight cycles were just as likely to stick to the study's diet and exercise plan. Anyone who stuck to the plan benefited.

78% eat breakfast every day.

75% weigh themselves at least once a week.

62% watch less than 10 hours of TV per week.

90% exercise, on average, about 1 hour per day

Assessing Your Weight

A high amount of body fat can lead to weight-related diseases and other health issues. Being underweight is also a health risk. Body Mass Index (BMI) and waist circumference are screening tools to estimate weight status in relation to potential disease risk. However, BMI and waist circumference are not diagnostic tools for disease risks. A trained healthcare provider should perform other health assessments to evaluate disease risk and diagnose disease status.

How to Measure and Interpret Weight Status

Adult Body Mass Index or BMI

BMI is a person's weight in kilograms divided by the square of height in meters. A high BMI can indicate high body fatness, and a low BMI can indicate too low body fatness. To calculate your BMI, see the BMI Calculator. Or determine your BMI by finding your height and weight in this BMI Index Chartexternal icon.

If your BMI is less than 18.5, it falls within the underweight range.

If your BMI is 18.5 to 24.9, it falls within the normal or Healthy Weight range.

If your BMI is 25.0 to 29.9, it falls within the overweight range.

If your BMI is 30.0 or higher, it falls within the obese range.

Weight that is higher than what is considered as a healthy weight for a given height is described as overweight or obese. Weight that is lower than what is considered as healthy for a given height is described as underweight.1

At an individual level, BMI can be used as a screening tool but is not diagnostic of the body fatness or health of an individual. A trained healthcare provider should perform appropriate health assessments in order to evaluate an individual's health status and risks.

How to Measure Height and Weight for BMI

Height and weight must be measured to calculate BMI. It is most accurate to measure height in meters and weight in kilograms. However, the BMI formula has been adapted for height measured in inches and weight measured in pounds. These measurements can be taken in a healthcare provider's office, or at home using a tape measure and scale.

Another way to estimate your potential disease risk is to measure your waist circumference. Excessive abdominal fat may be serious because it places you at greater risk for developing obesity-related conditions, such as Type 2 Diabetes, high blood pressure, and coronary artery disease. Your waistline may be telling you that you have a higher risk of developing obesity-related conditions if you are1:

A man whose waist circumference is more than 40 inches

A non-pregnant woman whose waist circumference is more than 35 inches

Waist circumference can be used as a screening tool but is not diagnostic of the body fatness or health of an individual. A trained healthcare provider should perform appropriate health assessments in order to evaluate an individual's health status and risks.

If you are what you eat, it follows that you want to stick to a healthy diet that's well balanced. "You want to eat a variety of foods," says Stephen Bickston, MD, AGAF, professor of internal medicine and director of the Inflammatory Bowel Disease Center at Virginia Commonwealth University Health Center in Richmond. "You don't want to be overly restrictive of any one food group or eat too much of another."

Healthy Diet: The Building Blocks

The best source of meal planning for most Americans is the U.S. Department of Agriculture (USDA) and U.S. Department of Health and Human Services Food Pyramid. The pyramid, updated in 2005, suggests that for a healthy diet each day you should eat:

6 to 8 servings of grains. These include bread, cereal, rice, and pasta, and at least 3 servings should be from whole grains. A serving of bread is one slice while a serving of cereal is 1/2 (cooked) to 1 cup (ready-to-eat). A serving of rice or pasta is 1/2 cup cooked (1 ounce dry). Save fat-laden baked goods such as croissants, muffins, and donuts for an occasional treat.

2 to 4 servings of fruits and 4 to 6 servings of vegetables. Most fruits and vegetables are naturally low in fat, making them a great addition to your healthy diet. Fruits and vegetables also provide the fiber, vitamins, and minerals you need for your body's systems to function at peak performance. Fruits and vegetables also will add flavor to a healthy diet. It's best to serve them fresh, steamed, or cut up in salads. Be sure to skip the calorie-laden toppings, butter, and mayonnaise, except on occasion. A serving of raw or cooked vegetables is equal to 1/2 cup (1 cup for leafy greens); a serving of a fruit is 1/2 cup or a fresh fruit the size of a tennis ball.

2 to 3 servings of milk, yogurt, and cheese. Choose dairy products wisely. Go for fat-free or reduced-fat milk or cheeses. Substitute yogurt for sour cream in many recipes and no one will notice the difference. A serving of dairy is equal to 1 cup of milk or yogurt or 1.5 to 2 ounces of cheese.

2 to 3 servings of meat, poultry, fish, dry beans, eggs, and nuts. For a healthy diet, the best ways to prepare beef, pork, veal, lamb, poultry, and fish is to bake or broil them. Look for the words "loin" or "round" in cuts of meats because they're the leanest. Remove all visible fat or skin before cooking, and season with herbs, spices, and fat-free marinades. A serving of meat, fish, or poultry is 2 to 3 ounces. Some crossover foods such as dried beans, lentils, and peanut butter can provide protein without the animal fat and cholesterol you get from meats. A ¼ cup cooked beans or 1 tablespoon of peanut butter is equal to 1 ounce of lean meat.

Use fats, oils, and sweets sparingly. No diet should totally eliminate any one food group, even fats, oils, and sweets. It's fine to include them in your diet as long as it's on occasion and in moderation, Bickston says.

Healthy Diet: Eat Right and the Right Amount

How many calories you need in a day depends on your sex, age, body type, and how active you are. Generally, active children ages 2 to 8 need between 1,400 and 2,000 calories a day. Active teenage girls and women can consume about 2,200 calories a day without gaining weight. Teenage boys and men who are very active should consume about 3,000 calories a day to maintain their weight. If you're not active, you calorie needs drop by 400 to 600 calories a day.

The best way to know how much to eat is to listen to your body, says Donald Novey, MD, an integrative medicine physician with the Advocate Medical Group in Park Ridge, Ill. "Pull away from the table when you're comfortable but not yet full. Wait about 20 minutes," he says. "Usually your body says, 'That's good.' If you're still hungry after that, you might want to eat a little more."

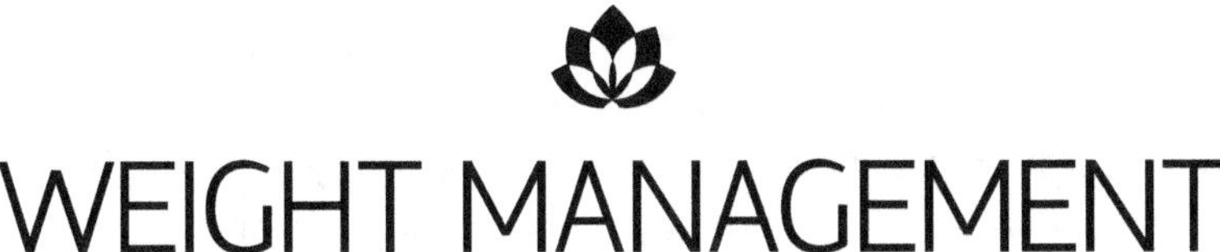

CHAPTER NINE

WEIGHT MANAGEMENT

The term 'weight management' refers to maintenance of one's weight within a healthy range, being neither overweight nor underweight. Overweight or obesity can be defined as an abnormal or excessive fat accumulation in our body. Overweight and obesity affect one's day to day physical performance. What is more important, these are major risk factors for heart disease, stroke, type II diabetes, osteoarthritis and certain forms of cancers. On the other hand, being underweight makes one vulnerable to gastrointestinal diseases and affects immune system adversely. Parents and teachers may please take note that as per World Health Organization (WHO) report, childhood obesity is associated with a higher chance of premature death and disability in adulthood1 . The problem of overweight is so huge and widespread that WHO has termed it 'global epidemic'. It is no longer confined to developed countries; it is increasing at faster rate in developing countries. As per WHO report, in 2005, globally approximately 1.6 billion adults (age 15+) were overweight and at least 400 million of them obese. However, the good news is that the problem of overweight and obesity is largely preventable. And, the solution lies in an intelligent mix of balanced diet, regular exercise and positive mind-set.

II. CAUSES OF OVERWEIGHT For a normal person who is not suffering from any medical abnormality, the fundamental cause of overweight and obesity is more caloric intake and less caloric expenditure. This caloric imbalance may occur due to following reasons – (i) Aging process – With age our body composition3 changes. There is an increase in fat percentage and decrease in fat free mass. Consequent to this, our Resting Metabolic Rate (RMR) declines. The decline in RMR means that our body now requires less number of calories for its maintenance. Failure to adjust our caloric intake to changed body composition leads to weight gain. (ii) Sedentary life style – Increasing urbanization, sedentary nature of work, widespread use of mechanized transport give us less scope for physical activity. Ignoring this fact and continuing with higher caloric intake contributes to weight gain. (iii) Discontinuation of exercise – Those earlier accustomed to regular physical exercise may suddenly discontinue exercise due to illness, work commitment or out of sheer laziness, yet continue with the usual high caloric intake. This would surely cause weight gain. It is not very uncommon to see many ex-sportspersons walking with those extra tyres of fat around their waist, for this reason only.(iv) Junk food – Frequent and indiscriminate consumption of junk foods is a major cause of overweight and obesity, especially among children. Junk foods are very high in calories due to their high contents of fats, sugar and salts. While high calories from fats and sugar directly contribute to weight gain, salt contributes so by causing more water retention in the body. (v) Poor understanding of exercise and nutrition – The relationship between amount of calories spent and calories gained has to be understood properly. Remember this simple common sense formula – for weight maintenance, caloric expenditure should be equal to caloric intake; for weight loss, caloric expenditure should be more than caloric intake and for weight gain, caloric expenditure should be less than caloric intake. Some of the new comers to exercise have a tendency to overestimate their energy expenditure during exercise and taking it as a licence to consume high calories food. This results into imbalance between caloric intake and caloric expenditure. III. WHAT IS THE IDEAL BODY WEIGHT (IBW) ? We are a generation obsessed with weight management. We are always in quest of an ideal body weight. We starve ourselves to ridiculous extent, put more faith in miracle machines, devour magic pills and spend thousands of rupees to visit slimming centres. The question is – what is the ideal body weight (IBW) for a person? The answer is – this is a WRONG question. In fact, there is NO ideal body weight for any one. From time to time, efforts have been made to devise some sort of Height-Weight Tables to determine IBW for a corresponding height. For 133 example, Metropolitan Life Insurance Height & Weight Table (1980), developed by Metropolitan Life Insurance Company, was based on data associated with long life of the subjects who were closer to average IBW. Later, Body Mass Index (BMI) came to be widely accepted as a simple, quick and convenient method for determination of overweight and obesity. BMI is calculated by dividing weight in kilograms by height in meters squared. BMI = 2 ( ) ( ) Height Mtr Weight Kg IBW is measured at a BMI between 18.5-24.99 Kg/m2 , overweight at a BMI of 25 kg/m2 or more and obesity at a BMI of 30 kg/m2 or more. These cut offs are based on association between BMI and chronic disease and mortality and have been adopted by the World Health Organization (WHO). Please see the following table – Classification of Overweight and Obesity by BMI Obesity class BMI kg.m2 Underweight < 18.5 Normal 18.5-24.9 Overweight 25.0-29.9 Obesity I 30.0-34.9 II 35.0-39.9 Extreme obesity III ≥40 However, despite its wide acceptability and use, the concept of BMI suffers from the following limitations: (i) BMI is not a valid4 method to assess body fat. It is based on a simplistic presumption that 'overweight' is due to excess fat and hence more the fat, greater the risk of diseases. Therefore, being 'overweight' is always undesirable. This presumption is not true. BMI lacks validity as it 4. Validity refers to the degree to which a test measures what it is supposed to measure. BMI cannot measure fat. 134 does not distinguish excess adiposity (fatness) from greater muscularity. In other words, it ignores the fact that overweight can also be caused by greater muscularity or a larger body frame. For example, sportspersons like bodybuilders, heavyweight boxers, footballers, sprinters etc. may be 'overweight' or even 'obese' by BMI standards despite their excellent athletic ability and low body fat percentage. There is a distinction between overweight due to excess fat and overweight due to excess muscularity. When your overweight is due to excess fat, it is a liability. It will reduce your physical performance and increase the risk of certain diseases. Such overweight is harmful, hence undesirable and a matter of concern. On the other hand, if your overweight is due to extra muscle gain, it will contribute to your better physical performance. Such overweight is useful hence desirable and a matter of celebration. Look at the following illustration– In above illustration BMI will blindly place both A and B in the same category. Whose health is more at risk? You cannot find any answer from BMI. Actually, in case of the person B, high % fat is a matter of concern while for A, low % fat and high % lean body mass is a matter of celebration though both of them have the same weight. (ii) BMI ignores the element of body frame size. A person of same height and body composition but of larger body frame may weigh more than his medium or small body frame counterpart. But for all three body frame sizes, the same IBW has been fixed. Thus when we prescribe the 135 same IBW for all body frame sizes and allow a concession of 10% (beyond which one would be categorized as overweight), it practically means allowing a narrower range of concession to a person of larger body frame (as he is already heavier due to his larger skeletal frame). This is not a fair practice.

Look at the following illustration – In this illustration D will have a greater BMI than C despite having equal % of body fat only because of his larger body frame. (iii) BMI is not a suitable measure of ideal weight in case of children. For adults who have stopped growing, BMI method presumes that thereafter an increase in their weight will by caused by an increase in their body fat. In case of children, their amount of body fat keeps on changing as they grow up. Their BMI may decrease during early school days (due to shedding of baby fat) and then again increase as they grow into adulthood (due to increased muscle mass and larger body frame). (iv) Similarly, BMI will underestimate the amount of body fat of an elderly person. I have found many persons declaring with satisfaction (and pride) that over the years they have maintained their ideal weight. Take example of a person who weighed 70 Kg at age of 20, 40 and 60. Look at the following illustration – 136 It is clear from this illustration that weight of the person has remained in an ideal weight range throughout despite increase in % body fat over the years (which is not a healthy sign). This person has lost muscle mass, bone mass and is still happy about his weight! By now, it must be fairly clear that it is not the 'overweight' as such but it is rather the 'over fat' which should be of our real concern. Now, the question arises – what is the ideal body fat (IBF)? IV. WHAT IS THE IDEAL BODY FAT (IBF)? Unfortunately, unlike Body Mass Index (BMI) there is no universally accepted set of body fat standards. Different studies have recommended for a minimal essential fat percentage of total body weight. Minimal fat is the body fat that is necessary for health. It is essential for our nervous system, cell membranes, regulation of body temperature and production of sex hormones. According to American College of Sports Medicine (ACSM), minimal fat percentage for men and women should be 5% and 10-12% of total body weight respectively5 . Body fat less than 10-12% in women may lead to bone-thinning disease osteoporosis. The healthy range of fat percentage may go upto 25% and 38% for men and women respectively6 . US Army standards allow upto 26% and 36% for men and women above 40 respectively7 . There are so many other studies which recommend an ideal fat % range with slight variations. Let's not embark upon this endless journey of finding 'the ideal body fat'. What is important for us is that we should be well within healthy range of body fat percentage. Lower the body fat percentage, the better will be our physical performance.

Well, this is the most intriguing part of the entire problem. Body fat can be measured by any of these methods, viz., Hydrostatic Weighing,

Air Displacement Plethysmography (ADP), Bioelectric Impedence Analysis (BIA), Ultrasound, Dual Energy Projection Method, Magnetic Resonance Imaging (MRI), Anthropometry (by measuring body parts, e.g., waist-hip ratio and skin fold calipers method). None of these methods is perfect and has its own limitations and error margin. Let the complexity of methods mentioned above for body fat measurement not worry you at all. I would suggest two rather simple methods which would help you to know about your health risks associated with body fat. These are – (i) Waist-Hip Ratio (WHR) – WHR is obtained by dividing the waist circumference by the hip circumference. For this, measure the smallest girth around your abdomen and the largest girth around your hips. (Don't cheat yourself by sucking in your belly to minimize your waist circumference!) (ii) Waist circumference (WC) – As mentioned above, waist circumference is to be obtained by measuring the smallest girth around your abdomen. Important for Indians – Studies have been conducted to determine cutoff values (for Indians) for BMI and upper-body adiposity (measured by Waist circumference) or WHR and their risk association with diabetes and cardiovascular disease. One such study found that universal criteria for BMI, WC or WHR did not hold good for all races. For a given BMI, Indians have higher upper-body adiposity and higher visceral fat when compared with the White population. This makes Indians more vulnerable for fat-related health risk at even lower BMI. Based on its findings, the study suggested that the healthy BMI for an Indian is <23 kg/m2 . Cut-off 138 values for WC are 85 cm for men and 80 cm for women. Cut-off values for WHR were 0.89 for men and 0.81 for women8 . The cut-off value for BMI may not be useful, when used in isolation to predict fat related health risk. However, cut-off values of WC and WHR are good predictor of one's health risks. V. METHODS OF WEIGHT (READ FAT) LOSS The underlying principle of a healthy fat loss programme is this – Lose fat but preserve your fat free mass (lean body mass). Never adopt a method which causes loss of muscle mass. We will discuss the following common methods of weight loss – A. By diet control only – Reduce total caloric intake and lose weight. This method is not recommended for the following reasons – (i) It ignores the basic principle of nutrition that our diet should be balanced – total calories-wise, ratio of nutrients-wise (i.e., 60% carbohydrate, 20% protein, 20% fat) and nutrition-wise (should have carbohydrates, proteins, fats, vitamins, minerals). In this method, one may simply cut the total amount of calories without paying any heed the quality of calories. This may lead to nutrition-specific health problems. (ii) In this method, generally the first victim of diet reduction is fat as fat is considered to be the main culprit causing overweight. One should not forget that inadequate fat intake would impair absorption of fatsoluble vitamins. (See section on Fats). (iii) You may not get enough proteins, carbohydrates and micronutrients. All this would result in lowered level of strength, energy, etc. (iv) One may be tempted to undertake 'crash dieting'. This is very harmful as well as a foolish method of weight loss. By crash diet one will surely lose weight but in the process he will also lose his muscles and health. It is foolish because in case of crash diet out body develops a 'starvation syndrome'. This syndrome is marked by a lowered Basal Metabolic Rate (BMI). If our body does not get enough calories, it develops a tendency to conserve energy by slowing down its systems and spending less energy on the same kind of activity. For example, an underfed runner will spend less amount of energy per mile compared to his 'prestarvation' phase. Thus at the end you don't gain much. B. By exercise only – Eat as usual, exercise more and lose weight. This method is also not recommended for the following reasons – (i) Without any diet control one may have to work out a lot, may be for hours every day. This may result in overtraining and injury. One may not have luxury of so much time also. (ii) One may be psychologically charged up and overestimate the amount of caloric expenditure during exercise. The worse, he may have a tendency to reward himself with more food after exercising! The end result will be weight gain only. C. By both diet control and exercise – Exercise more, eat less and lose weight. This is the healthiest and most lasting method of fat loss. However, it is not recommended to lose more than 500 gms weight per week. Unless you are going to participate in some weight category specific sport, go slow. This method will ensure that your health and fitness never gets compromised in the process of weight loss. Rapid weight loss affects immune system, reduces muscle strength and glycogen level and adversely affects physical performance. Important– (i) Interestingly, it may happen that once you are into serious strength training, you may actually gain weight due to gain in your muscle mass. 140 Don't be alarmed by this. This is healthy weight gain. Be happy and celebrate this weight gain! (ii) Take up activities which burn more energy in less time. For example, running will burn more energy than walking. Running on a hill will burn more energy than running on a track. In short, all activities performed at higher intensity and for longer duration will burn more energy. (iii) Initially, minimum caloric intake per day should not be less than 1800 – 2000 kcal which is required for maintenance of our body system. (iv) Did you ever wonder why during recent years your body fat percentage increased even though you maintained the same exercise routine and ate the same amount of food? The fact is that as you age, your body undergoes certain irreversible changes. Adults lose about 0.2 kg of muscle per year during their 30s and 40s. This process is known as sarcopenia. The rate of muscle loss increases to 0.45 kg in their 50s and 60s9 . With decreased muscle mass your caloric needs will also decrease as muscles consume more calories. If you continue with the same amount of food, extra calories will be now stored as fat and will add to your weight. Therefore, bring changes in your diet accordingly, and take less calories as you age. Exercise combined with adequate diet will reduce the process of sarcopenia. (v) Decrease dietary fat. However, do not go to the other extreme. Severe restriction of fats may deprive your body of some vital fat-soluble vitamins (see chapter on Fats). (vi) Your choice of food should be such that it gives less calories but has high nutrients. For example, vegetables, fruits, salads, soups are low calorie foods, but very high in vitamins and minerals. The diet should provide variety of foods, high in nutrition and low in calories.

(vii) Be comfortable with your age, exercise and food. If you no longer enjoy your exercise or food, it is time to stop and review your routine. It is quite possible that you are overtraining or over-restraining yourself. Remember, both exercise and food have very wide ranging psychological implications. You will not gain much, rather you will harm yourself, by sticking to a regimen of exercise and food that allows you no stimulation or satisfaction. VI. SWEATING AND WEIGHT LOSS It will not be out of place to mention here that there are many among us who innocently believe that the more they sweat, the more they would lose fat. The fact is that there is no relation between sweating and fat loss. Sweating is just a cooling mechanism of the body. It brings out water and salts, not fat. Had there been any relationship between sweating and fat loss, there would have been more number of cozy sauna baths in the world than the gyms with their monstrous equipments! The mother nature always favours only those who believe in hard (and harder) work (outs)! Weight loss caused by sweating is a false and temporary weight loss. This is actually a loss of body fluid. Firstly, one should not dehydrate himself to 'lose weight' as there are many harmful effects of dehydration. Secondly, the moment fluid is replenished, one would regain original weight. VII. EATING DISORDERS Eating disorders originate from an individual's distorted self body image.

Studies have shown that these disorders are more prevalent among adolescents and young women, who are highly conscious of the shape and size of their body. Skinny models, cinema idols, dolls, etc. reinforce the idea among these vulnerable sections of the population that 'thin is beautiful'. 142 These are the characteristics of a person who is vulnerable to eating disorders. He/she – ? Feels herself fat even though people tell that she is thin. ? Worries too much about what to eat and what not to. ? Rushes to weighing machine to check weight after every party night. ? Avoids friends' company and eats alone. He/she gets anxious when invited to eat. ? Gets depressed when an exercise session is missed. ? Swears not to eat this food or that food. Anorexia Nervosa The term literally means 'loss of hunger on a psychological basis'. In this condition the person, though hungry, stops eating for fear of gaining fat and starts to starve. There are two types of anorexia – a) Restricting type – In this type the kind and amount of food is severely restricted; b) Binge eating/purging type – In this type one firstly eats the food and then throws it out by spitting, vomiting, using laxatives or enema. Warning signs of anorexia include rapid loss of weight, obsession with weight, obsession with exercise, sensitivity to cold, decline in work/ school performance, growth of baby-fine hair over face and body, dry hair/ skin, yellowish skin, irregular menstrual periods, constipation, abnormally slow pulse rate at rest. 143 Bulimia Nervosa Bulimia nervosa is binge-eating followed by purging. Binge eating is uncontrolled, eating of abnormally high amounts of food. Then comes 'purging' stage. Purging is done by use of laxatives, enema or vomiting to get rid of 'excess' food. Some persons prefer fasting or doing heavy exercise to 'compensate' for the excess food eaten. VIII. WEIGHT GAIN The problem of desirable weight gain by underweight individuals is the other end of the problem of weight management. Some of the commonly used methods for weight gain are – A. Exercise and diet – An increase in intensity and volume of exercise, especially, resistance training, (e. g. weight training) causes muscle hypertrophy (muscle gain). When combined with increased intake of diet, especially protein, it results into a healthy weight gain. B. Protein and Amino Acids supplements – An increase in the intake of protein above the RDA (.8gm/kg body weight) helps to gain muscle mass. But excess of protein intake has its own harmful implications. This issue has been elaborately discussed in the section on Proteins. C. Creatine supplements – Creatine monohydrate loading is popular among athletes. This results into an increase in body mass (1-2 kg) during a week. However, it is yet to be determined whether this increase in weight is due to increased lean muscle tissue or increased water retention. Moreover, prolonged intake of creatine causes overloading of kidneys by nitrogen worsening of allergy problems, disturbance of insulin functions, dehydration. D. Anabolic steroids – Through a very popular method among unscrupulous athletes to gain muscularity, it is fraught with many dangers. Some of the dangers of use of steroid are – reductions in the high density 144 lipoprotein cholesterol (HDL), increase in low density lipoprotein (LDL) cholesterol, low testosterone production and atrophy of the testes, liver damage, risk of cardiovascular disease, etc. With prolonged use of steroid men develop women-like features and vice versa in voice, facial hair, breasts, etc. Recommended Method for Weight Gain Combining resistance training with an increase in total dietary calories will provide a safe, systematic and sure way to weight gain. A slight increase in the protein intake above the RDA has been found to be very effective in gaining more lean muscle mass. IX. EXERCISE AND WEIGHT CONTROL Weight control as such is a complex phenomenon. The problem of overweight or underweight is not simply a calculation of daily food intake and energy expenditure. Various studies have been undertaken and experiments carried out on different samples of people to ascertain the relationship between caloric intake and caloric expenditure. However, the results have not always been uniform. In our daily life also we find many examples around us. Some of our friends refuse to lose weight despite their pitiably meagre food intake while there are also the gifted ones who binge on every food they get and still maintain their enviably lean body frame. One explanation given for this anomalous behaviour of human body is that genetic factors play predominant role in determination of our body composition. Another study suggests that the body maintains a certain size of fat cells. Beyond a limit, fat cell size cannot be reduced irrespective of amount of food or duration of exercise. Difference in resting metabolic rates (RMR) is also one of the factors that explains this anomaly. Between two individuals there is always a difference in the amount of energy they actually derive and store from the food or in the amount of energy they need to maintain their weight. With equal food intake and equal amount of 145 exercise a person with higher RMR (who spends more energy) will gain less weight than a person with lower RMR (who spends less energy). However, things cannot be left upon genetics alone. There are certain definite ways in which exercise helps weight control – (i) Intense and prolonged exercise elevates metabolic rate for some time after exercise.

This means that our body would spend more energy on the same activity even after exercise. (ii) Exercise also increases thermogenic effect of food eaten. This means that you would spend more energy to process the food. (iii) Exercise increases lean body mass. Lean body mass includes muscles, bone, water. Muscles require more energy. This means that a more muscular man would burn more energy. How Fat Burns? Fats are basically fuel stored in our body for hard times like starvation. Initially, it is mostly the carbohydrate which is utilized by the body for energy. But after 30-40 minutes of continuous exercise fat will be utilized more and carbohydrates less for energy. Better conditioning through exercise (both aerobic and anaerobic) helps the body burn fat in the following way – (i) Aerobic exercise in particular enhances the development of capillaries to the muscles. This means more blood supply and thereby more oxygen to the muscles. With more blood flow and greater oxygen supply fat is more efficiently burnt. (ii) During aerobic exercise and after anaerobic exercise, considerable mobilization of free fatty acids occurs. Free fatty acids oxidation is related to body fat losses. (iii) Prolonged, low-intensity aerobic activities e.g., slow jogging, cycling are more effective ways to burn fat, as fat burns only as long as oxygen is available. 146 X. SOME PRACTICAL TIPS FOR IDEAL FAT MANAGEMENT (i) Change your lifestyle. Grab every opportunity to walk, jog, exercise. (ii) Never starve. You will have a tendency to overeat or eat indiscriminately after starvation. (iii) Take fruits between meals as snack. Avoid fast food. Fast food will make you slow. (iv) Keep healthy snacks of your choice ready at hand. (v) Reduce total fat consumption. Shift from saturated fats to unsaturated fats. (vi) Consume less sugar. (vii) Do at least 30-40 minutes of moderate to high intensity activity on most of the days of the week. (viii) Enjoy your food. Let's confess it – junk foods are tasty, often tastier than 'health' foods. Most of the children will agree with me. Once in a while it is all right to enjoy junk food. But let us eat it in a 'healthier' manner. Mothers may add more greens and less fat in the junk foods for enhancing their nutritive value. Finally, throw away the weighing machine out of your house. That is the real junk lying in your mind and scaring you for such a long time. Remember that focus on weight loss is a misplaced focus. Instead, focus on your gains in health and fitness. If you are getting better and better everyday as far as your health, fitness and satisfaction is concerned, you don't have to worry about your weight at all.

CHAPTER TEN

Special Exercises for Special People

Fitness isn't only for those buff, 20-something gyms gods. In fact, you can start exercising in your 80s and still reap the benefits of a healthier, longer life. And the earlier in life you start working out, the more likely it will become a lifelong habit. Chapter 23 offers some tips and advice for beginning an exercise program in your senior years. How early is early enough? How about the womb? One study shows that women who exercise during pregnancy have leaner babies who turn into leaner kids. The benefits aren't only for the kids, however. From reducing back pain and encouraging better sleep patterns to encountering an easier delivery to slipping back into your old jeans more quickly, exercising during pregnancy offers incredible health benefits. See Chapter 21 for a short tutorial on getting and staying fit during pregnancy. For an in-depth look at pregnancy workouts, check out Fit Pregnancy For Dummies by Catherine Cram and Tere Stouffer Drenth (published by Wiley). Kids, perhaps more than any other age group, understand that being active is fun. If you can tap into their natural love of activities, especially games, sports, and dancing, you can help your kids avoid the alarming rates of obesity that plague children today. Without emphasizing "exercise" or "workouts," you can introduce your child to all sorts of healthy activities that encourage a lifelong fitness. Keep the emphasis on fun, without pushing your child into competitions or activities she doesn't enjoy, and you'll help your child become an adult with a strong body and a healthy heart.We've never been fond of tests that you can't study for. Nevertheless, we think the first step toward getting in shape is having your fitness evaluated. Don't panic. This test isn't like your driver's license renewal exam: You can't flunk, and you don't have to stand in line for three hours listening to people rant and rave about government bureaucracy. A fitness test simply gives you key information about your physical condition. We constantly hear people say, "I'm so out of shape. I need to lose weight." But that's like telling a travel agent, "I'm in Europe. I need to go to Africa." Your travel agent needs to know the specifics: Are you in Rome? Berlin? Moscow? Do you want to go to Cairo? Cape Town? The Kalahari Desert? Before you embark on a fitness program, you need to know your starting point with the same sort of precision. A fitness evaluation gives you important departure information, such as your heart rate, body fat, strength, and flexibility. Armed with these facts, you or your trainer can design an intelligent plan to get you to your fitness destination. And when you get there, you'll have the numbers to prove just how far you've come.When you join a gym, one of the first things you should be asked to do — after signing your check, of course — is to fill out a health-history questionnaire. Your answers to these questions give a snapshot of your overall wellbeing, including your eating and exercise habits, your risk for developing cardiovascular disease, and any orthopedic limitations or medical conditions that you may have. Typical questions include: Do you have any chronic joint problems such as arthritis? Do you have a high stress level? Are you currently taking any over-the-counter or prescription medications? If you don't belong to a gym, ask yourself the following questions, which are designed to indicate your risk of developing heart disease: Are you inactive? Do you have a history of heart disease? Do you have diabetes or high blood sugar? Do you have a history of high blood pressure? Did your mother, father, sister, or brother develop any form of heart disease before age 50? Do you smoke cigarettes, or have you quit within the last two years? Do you have high cholesterol — either total cholesterol higher than 200 mg/dl or HDL less than 40 mg/dl? If you answer "yes" to at least one question and you're over age 35, see a physician for a complete medical evaluation before you even pursue a fitness testing session. A physician is the only one who can accurately determine whether exercising puts you in any danger. If you answer "yes" to two or more questions, get a checkup no matter how old you are. Some gyms request that you be tested by a physician if a staff member feels you may have a medical problem. Don't groan; a request like this indicates that your gym is on the ball. Some health clubs just want your money. They may not require any testing — other than the test that determines whether you can sign your name on a credit-card slip. If that's the case, you need to take responsibility for getting tested. After you fill out your questionnaire, your tester should discuss the answers with you and ask for more information if necessary. If you're a smoker, for example, he may ask you how much you smoke. Respond honestly and thoroughly. Don't say that you run 5 miles a day if you haven't broken a sweat since high school — or if you intend to run every day but just haven't gotten around to it.Your heart rate, also known as your pulse, is the number of times your heart beats per minute. Your fitness evaluation should include a measure of your resting heart rate — your heart rate when you're sitting still. Ideally, your resting heart rate should be between 60 and 90 beats per minute. It may be slower if you're fit or genetically predisposed to a low heart rate; it may be faster if you're nervous or have recently downed three double cappuccinos. In addition to caffeine, stress and certain medications can speed up your heart rate. To be sure, take your heart rate first thing in the morning for three consecutive days and find the average to determine your heart rate. After a month or two of regular exercise, your resting heart rate usually drops. This means that your heart has become more efficient. It may need to beat only 80 times per minute to pump the same amount of blood (or more) than it used to pump in 90 beats. In the long run, this saves wear and tear on your heart.Have a professional test your blood pressure. Home blood-pressure machines tend to be inaccurate, as do those contraptions in the mall that charge a quarter for a reading. Blood pressure is a measurement of how open your blood vessels are. Low numbers mean that your heart doesn't have to work very hard to pump the blood through your blood vessels. Ideally, your blood pressure should read 115/75 or below, a lower standard than the old standby of 120/80. If it's slightly higher, don't get stressed (that only increases it even more). However, if your blood pressure is higher than 140/90, you are considered hypertensive, a fancy term for having high blood pressure. In case you're wondering, the top number, called your systolic blood pressure, measures pressure as your heart ejects blood. The bottom number, your diastolic blood pressure, measures pressure when your heart relaxes and prepares for its next pump. If you get a high blood-pressure reading, ask your tester to try again. The numbers can be affected by many factors, such as illness, caffeine, nervousness, or racing into your test because you were late. But if you repeatedly get high readings, see a doctor.

How Much of You Is Fat? During your evaluation, your tester will probably weigh you. Just know that your weight is of limited value. When you hop on a scale, you learn the grand total weight of your bones, organs, blood, fat, muscle, and other tissues. This number can be misleading because muscle weighs more per square inch than fat. Consider two men who stand 5'8" and weigh 190 pounds. One guy may be a lean bodybuilder who has a lot of muscle packed onto his frame. Another guy may be a couch potato whose gut hangs 4 inches over his belt buckle. Even a low weight doesn't necessarily indicate good health or fitness. It may simply mean that you have small bones and little muscle. More helpful than your body weight is your body composition — how much of your body is composed of fat and how much is composed of everything else. Your body composition is also called your body-fat percentage. If you score a 25 percent on a fat test, this means that 25 percent of your weight is composed of fat. Like your weight, your body-fat percentage is not necessarily a measure of your health. True, cardiovascular disease, diabetes, and certain cancers are more prevalent among overweight people — men who have more than about 20 percent body fat and women who have more than about 30 percent body fat. However, some researchers believe that these health problems are not caused by the extra fat itself but rather by a lack of exercise and a poor diet. In other words, if you exercise regularly and eat well, extra body fat may not compromise your health. So consider your body-fat score in a context with other health measures, such as your cholesterol levels, blood pressure, and other gauges of fitness, such as a submaximal test and your resting heart rate. An additional number to consider is the circumference of your waist. Excess abdominal fat — the type that lies deep in your belly, clumped around your organs — is linked to increased risk for heart disease. Heavy thighs, on the other hand, do not appear to be related to health problems. (In other words — to use terms we can all relate to — a beer belly is more harmful to your health than saddlebags.) Men with waist measurements greater than 40 and women with waist measurements greater than 35 should consult a physician. Although body fat testing has its limits, your results can give you great insight into how your fat-loss and exercise program is coming along. Sure, your scale can tell you that you lost 7 pounds. But a body-fat test can tell you that your 7-pound loss means that you lost 10 pounds of fat and gained 3 pounds of muscle, results that are probably more motivating.

Body-fat testing also can tell you if you have too little fat. Maybe you can never be too rich, but you definitely can be too thin. For women, super-low body fat — below about 16 percent — may lead to problems such as irregular menstrual periods, permanent bone loss, and a high rate of bone fractures. Keep in mind that every body-fat testing method has room for error. At a recent fitness convention, Suzanne had her body fat measured by two different methods — and appeared to have gained 11 percent body fat in a matter of 15 minutes. You may even get wildly different readings using the same test, depending on the skill of the tester or the condition of the equipment. The only way to measure body fat with complete accuracy is to burn yourself up and take a carbon count of the ashes. Because that technique doesn't draw too many volunteers, scientists have developed a number of other methods. Here's a look at the ones you're most likely to come across.

The most common body-fat test uses the skinfold caliper, a gizmo that resembles a stun gun with salad tongs attached (see Figure 2-1). When your tester fires, the tongs pinch your skin, pulling your fat away from your muscles and bones. (You feel moderate discomfort, like when your great aunt pinches your cheek on the holidays.) Typically, the tester pinches three to seven different sites on your body, such as your abdomen, the back of your arm, and the back of your shoulder. The thickness of each pinch is plugged into a formula to determine your body-fat percentage. Your tester should pinch each site two or three times to verify the measurement. Many things can go wrong with a caliper test. The tester may not pinch exactly the right spot, or he may not pull all the fat away from the bone. Or he may pinch too hard and accidentally yank some of your muscle. Also, research suggests that certain formulas are more accurate for certain ethnic groups, age ranges, and fitness levels. Experts give this test a margin of error of four points, meaning your actual body-fat percentage could be four points higher or lower than it actually is. Be sure to get tested before your workout. When you exercise, blood travels to your skin to cool you down. This can cause your skin to swell, and you may test fatter than you really are. Plus, calipers can slip if your skin is wet from sweat.

How Strong Are You? Fear not: You won't be required to do one-arm push-ups or lift a barbell that weighs more than your dad. Strength tests, like the other tests that we describe in this chapter, are simply designed to give you a starting point. If you get started on a good weight-lifting program and stick to it, you're likely to see dramatic changes when you take another fitness test in two or three months. Most health clubs don't take true strength measurements; in other words, they don't measure the absolute maximum amount of weight you're capable of lifting. Going for your "max" can be dangerous and can cause more than a little muscle soreness. Instead, gyms test your muscular endurance: how many times you can move a much lighter weight. You can do many of these tests at home. Having a friend count for you and make sure you're doing the exercise correctly is a help. Here are some common muscular endurance measures. Measuring your upper-body strength Count how many push-ups you can do without stopping or losing good form. For this test, men do military push-ups, with their legs out straight and toes on the floor. Women do modified push-ups, with their knees bent and feet off the floor. Lower your entire body at once until your upper arms are parallel to the floor. Pull your abdominals in to prevent your back from sagging. Do this test correctly! One guy we watched didn't have the strength to lower his body all the way, so he just bobbed his head up and down.

Whatever your goals are, keeping track of your workouts in a workout log (also called a workout diary or training diary) can help you get better results. You can look back at the end of each week and say, "I did that?" And you may be inspired to accomplish even more. Keeping a log shows you whether your goals are realistic and gives you insight into your exercise patterns. If you're losing weight, building strength, or developing stamina, you won't have to wonder what works, because you'll have a blow-by-blow description of everything you've done to reach your goals. On the other hand, if you get injured or stuck in a rut, you can turn to your diary for clues as to why. You may discover that if you don't eat before you cycle, you cover your usual route five minutes slower. Maybe you pull a hamstring every time you run over a certain hilly course. Maybe you're more susceptible to catching a cold if you don't rest at least one day each week. A workout diary keeps you honest. You may think that you're working out four times a week. But when you flip through your log, you may realize that you've been overestimating your efforts. Bookstores and sporting-goods stores carry a variety of logs, some aimed at walkers, others at weight lifters; others have space to chart any activity you can think of. You also can buy nifty computer software to monitor your progress or use a Web-based tracking program. In Chapter 25, we mention some of our favorite products for recording your workouts. You can also use (photocopying the page) to see whether you enjoy tracking your workouts on paper.

Walk into a health club or fitness-equipment store and you're likely to encounter rows of high-tech contraptions that appear to be part video game, part escalator, and part lawn mower. Don't be alarmed. The consoles of these machines may resemble the control panel of Apollo 13, but with a little help, even a rookie can understand all the flashing red dots and beeping green arrows. Be thankful for all this technology because it makes indoor aerobic exercise a lot more fun than it used to be. For all your sweat, the screen offers you instant gratification — the number of miles that you walk, steps that you climb, minutes that you cycle, and calories that you burn. Cardiovascular machines tend to come and go. Since the first edition of this book, we've seen the rise and fall of various riders, gliders, and skaters. So we're not going to give you a rundown of every crazy invention that's made its way onto an infomercial. Instead, this chapter covers the solid, proven machines, such as treadmills, rowers, bikes, and stair-climbers, as well as a relative newcomer that we believe is here to stay: the elliptical trainer. We tell you how to take the drudgery out of exercising in place and how to position your body on each machine so that you burn the most calories and avoid injury At the gym one day, Suzanne was pumping away on the stair-climber next to a very fit woman. For a brief moment, the woman looked away from her machine to say hello to a friend. When she looked back, her 45-minute workout had ended, and she had missed the final calorie readout. Horrified, the woman uttered several curse words and then stormed into the locker room — as if not knowing her exact calorie burn negated the entire 45 minutes of effort. That may be an extreme case, but most of us do get a psychological boost from knowing how many calories we just burned. There's just one problem: The information may not be accurate. For the most part, the formulas used to calculate calories burned are derived from tests done on healthy young males — and in some cases, elite athletes working near their maximum effort. This does not always translate accurately for the rest of us. For instance, a recent study conducted found that fitness equipment readouts may overestimate calorie count for obese women by as much as 80 calories for 30 minutes of moderate intensity walking. Other research has found that calorie predictions are skewed even further if you lean your body weight against the handrails, grip tightly, or otherwise position your body on a machine in a way that makes the exercise less strenuous. Some studies have shown that calculations can be off by as much as 50 percent. Sometimes it's not the formulas or your technique that skew the calorie count; it's the deceptive marketing strategy of the machine's manufacturer. A researcher for one cardio-equipment manufacturer admitted to us that his company intentionally boosts the calorie information by as much as 30 percent so that people may, subconsciously, prefer their machines over other brands.

We suspect that elliptical machines (described in the "Elliptical trainer" section later in this chapter) have particularly generous calorie readouts. Case in point: When Liz does a fairly easy elliptical workout, the machine tells her that she burns 12 calories per minute — a number that seems suspiciously high. In fact, in order to achieve the same calorie burn on the treadmill (known to be an accurate machine), she needs to run at a brisk 8 mph, a pace that shoots her heart rate way up into the huff-and-puff zone. We're skeptical that these two workouts are equivalent. The most accurate machines tend to be the treadmill and the stationary bike because the contraptions have been so well studied. In recent years, stairclimbers have adjusted calorie estimates drastically downward to better reflect reality.

It's no coincidence that "treadmill" is listed under "tedium" in Roget's Thesaurus; imitating a laboratory rodent is not among life's thrills. No matter what type of exercise machine you use and no matter how many flashing dots you're rewarded with, boredom is bound to hit you at some point. In this section, we suggest ways to divert your attention so that your 20, 30, or 40 minutes pass before you know it. Eventually, you may actually begin to enjoy the sensations of sweat and fatigue, and using these machines won't seem like a chore. Take a cardio-machine class It used to be that if you wanted a cardio workout in the company of a perky instructor and enthusiastic classmates, you had to take step aerobics or some type of dance class. But now the group-exercise concept includes machines, too. The trend started with indoor cycling classes known as spinning or studio cycling and has since expanded to treadmills, stair-climbers, and rowing machines. Group cycling has become so popular that most new clubs now build separate rooms for these classes. (See Chapter 4 for more details about group cycling.) Treadmill classes that go by the name of Treading and Trekking are also catching on. Concept II, a top rowing machine brand, has developed a half-hour group class called Boathouse, and StairMaster has introduced a 20-minute climbing class called Stomp. Instructors of these cardio classes guide you through a workout as if you're running, climbing, or rowing outdoors. You imagine bounding up pristine mountain hills, sprinting through meadows, or finishing the Tour de France. A good instructor can make the experience so much fun that you almost forget you're in a room with a dozen other stinky, sweaty people going absolutely nowhere. Vary your workouts If you don't want to take a class or you work out at home, you can make your workouts more entertaining simply by varying your pace. Most machines have a manual mode that allows you to control the intensity of the workout. Chapter 9: Using Cardio Machines 129 You push one arrow to speed up the pace, another to slow it down. Use the manual mode to design your own workouts, incorporating the training techniques that we describe in Chapter 8. You should also experiment with the various programs already entered in the computer's memory. These programs are great because you don't have to decide what to do next. Most programs have built-in warm-up and cooldown periods; in between, you vary your pace. For instance, many machines offer a random program; every 10 to 30 seconds, the machine surprises you by changing the tension. Most treadmills offer programs like "A Romp in the Park," which may be a 3-mile walk or jog over rolling hills. The treadmill automatically inclines and declines during these workouts. Listen to music or a book on tape Rock, rap, pop, or country — go with whatever gets your adrenaline pumping. If Shania Twain works for you, so be it. A tape that mixes fast and slow songs can add variety to your workout, because your pace tends to be in sync with the music. One study showed that women who exercised to music lasted 25 percent longer than those who worked out in silence. At some gyms you can plug your headphones into a system that offers dozens of CD selections and audio channels. Or try listening to a book on tape. You may prefer to get wrapped up in a good story or learn how to manage your love life. If you rely on a tape or CD player to keep you going, make sure that you keep a load of extra batteries in your gym bag. We can't count the times we've shown up at the gym with our tape players only to find that the batteries are dead — along with our motivation. At some gyms, you can listen to music without the need for batteries, or even a tape or CD player. At these clubs, the cardio machines are equipped with high-tech systems: Attached to each treadmill, bike, or other machine is a tape and CD player, along with a small TV screen that even offers Internet access. The only catch is you have to buy special wireless headphones that cost up to $100. These systems require you to bring your own headphones and plug them into a small box attached to the machine. Or, you need your own personal stereo and must tune into an FM frequency to pick up the various TV stations.Kill two birds with one stone: Burn calories while you catch up on your reading. Suzanne is a much more informed citizen during the winter, when she spends a fair amount of time on the stair-climber, than she is during the summer, when she's outside on her road bike. This is a good time to read the fitness magazines we talk about in the Appendix. Exercise magazines offer lots of encouragement and tend to contain easy-to-skim lists. When you're drenched in sweat on the elliptical trainer, taking in "Ten Ways to Boost Energy and Get Stronger" is a lot easier than concentrating on an essay about Indonesian politics. Note: As we explain in the "Treadmill" section later in this chapter, don't read while you're walking or running on the treadmill. Exercise in short spurts To break up the monotony, do ten minutes on the treadmill, followed by ten minutes on the bike, and then ten minutes on the rowing machine. Or try short bouts on a cardio machine with five minutes of weight lifting. As we explain in Chapter 8, it's a myth that you must exercise for 20 or 30 consecutive minutes. Breaking up your workout into small chunks isn't a good strategy to use every day if you're training for a marathon, but if your goal is simply to burn calories and improve your health, the total time you spend exercising is what matters most. Think, but not too hard People tend to have their most creative ideas when they're doing something repetitive that doesn't involve their mind completely. But don't set out to solve the U.S. health-care crisis during your workout. Instead, use your time Chapter 9: Using Cardio Machines 131 to ponder more solvable dilemmas, like how you can get your boss off your back. You may even want to keep a tape recorder handy, in case a flash of brilliance comes along. Monitor your heart rate To keep yourself occupied, use a heart-rate monitor to create an interval program. For instance, after warming up, alternate five minutes at the low end of your target zone with five minutes at the high end.Many machines have heart-rate monitors built into them. Your heart rate registers when you grasp the handles. Or, you can wear a strap around your chest; the machine picks up the signal from the strap and beams it to the console so that your heart rate is displayed right alongside your speed and distance. The strap is more accurate than the handles, but you do have to bring your own heart-rate-monitor chest strap from home, if your gym doesn't provide them.

can't stand. Some people find the treadmill invigorating; others consider it more tedious than peeling potatoes. We suggest you try all the machines at your gym or at an equipment store before you buy one. No single cardio machine is better than the rest. What matters most is how often you use the thing. No matter what machine you use, always keep a water bottle and a towel within reach. Many gym machines have water bottle holders, and you can buy them cheaply for your home equipment. Also, stay tuned to how your 132 Part III: Getting to the Heart of the Matter body feels. If your knee hurts or you start to feel faint, don't ignore the pain or try to drown it out by cranking up the volume on your stereo headphones. You may be damaging muscles or joints. That said, here's a look at the most popular cardiovascular machines. Treadmill Treadmills are the motorized equivalent of walking or running in place. You simply keep up with a belt that's moving under your feet. Treadmill workouts burn about the same number of calories as walking or running outdoors. The only exception seems to be running uphill. When you incline the treadmill to simulate running uphill, it's somewhat easier than running up real-life hills of the same grade. But walking uphill on a treadmill is virtually the same as walking uphill outdoors. Who will like it Treadmills are especially popular in crowded cities, where you need to be part cutting horse, part smog filter to run or walk through the streets. Treadmills are great for beginners because they require little coordination to use. Plus, treadmills can move at a slow enough pace to accommodate even the most out-of-shape exercisers. People with back pain, bad knees, or weak ankles often find treadmills kinder to their joints than concrete or cement. Today's treadmills are springier and more shock-absorbing than ever. Many have added flashy new features, such as Internet hookups so that you can run and walk with other treadmillers from all over the globe. Some treadmills can store up to 100 personal programs. Who will hate it You need a very strong or very blank mind to do long workouts on a treadmill. Most people find more than a half-hour on this machine mind-numbing, even with entertainment. If you crave the wind whipping through your hair and scenery flashing by, reserve the treadmills for emergency aerobic situations only. Running also places more impact on your joints than most other exercises and may not be a favorite if you have a bad lower back, achy knees, or weak ankles. Treadmill user tips Treadmills are among the easiest cardio machines to use. Still, treadmill users are not immune to poor posture. And if you're not paying attention, you can stumble. On occasion you may see someone slide off the treadmill like a can of beans on a supermarket conveyor belt. Here are some tips to make sure this doesn't happen to you: Chapter 9: Using Cardio Machines 133 Start slowly. Most treadmills have safety features that prevent them from starting out at breakneck speeds, but don't take any chances. Always place one foot on either side of the belt as you turn on the machine, and step on the belt only after you determine that it's moving at the slow set-up speed, usually between 1 and 2 miles per hour. Don't rely on the handrails. Holding on for balance when you learn how to use the machine is okay, but let go as soon as you feel comfortable. You move more naturally if you swing your arms freely. You're working at too high a level if you have to imitate a water-skier — in other words, if you hold onto the front rails and lean back. This is a common phenomenon among people who incline the treadmill, and this position is bad news for your elbows and for the machine. Plus, you're not fooling anyone; you're burning far fewer calories than the readout indicates. However, if you have balance issues, go ahead and grasp the handrails lightly so that you feel steady and secure. Look straight ahead. Your feet tend to follow your eyes, so if you focus on what's in front of you, you usually walk straight ahead instead of veering off to the side. When you're in the middle of a workout and someone calls your name, don't turn around to answer. This piece of advice may seem obvious now, but wait until it happens to you. Expect to feel disoriented. The first few times you use a treadmill, you may feel dizzy when you step off. Your body is just wondering why the ground suddenly stopped moving. Don't worry. Most people only experience this vertigo once or twice. Never go barefoot. Always wear a good pair of walking or running shoes for your treadmill workout. Don't read on the treadmill. You risk losing your balance and stumbling off the side or back.

Fresh air: What a concept. With all the hoopla these days about space-age, indoor exercise contraptions, it's easy to forget you can get a great workout in the great outdoors. You may even get a better workout — burning more calories per minute — because outdoor activities sometimes involve more muscles than their indoor counterparts. For example, when you park yourself on a stationary bicycle, your upper-body muscles basically get a free ride — you can easily read a magazine as you pedal away. But when you take your bike out for a spin, your chest, arm, abdominal, and back muscles are all called up for active duty. In this chapter, we cover some of the most popular and invigorating outdoor aerobic activities. We discuss what gear you need and how much it costs, and we offer training strategies and safety tips for rookies and klutzes alike. Walking Can you really get fit by walking? Absolutely — as long as you walk long enough, hard enough, and often enough. (If you're asking, "How long?", "How hard?", and "How often?", check out Chapter 8.) A recent study found that, among people who are successful in maintaining long-term weight loss, nearly 80 percent walk as their main physical activity. The beauty of walking is, it's simply a matter of putting one foot in front of the other. Sure, walking burns fewer calories per minute than jogging, but most people last longer on a walk than a run, so you can make up for the deficit. Plus, compared to runners, walkers enjoy a relatively low injury rate. However, we're not going to sugar-coat this: Some exercisers find walking to be a big, fat bore. Suzanne hates walking so much that she'll spend 15 minutes searching for a good parking space at her gym before a one-hour workout on the stationary bike. (She can't help it; she grew up in Los Angeles, where you drive to visit your next-door neighbor.) Essential walking gear Although the rest of the animal kingdom does fine without the benefit of special equipment, human feet don't have adequate padding to meet the demands of walking in the modern world. You need a good pair of walking shoes to avoid foot, ankle, knee, hip, and lower-back problems. Expect to spend at least $50 for good walking shoes, which should hold up for 1,000 to 1,500 miles. (Running shoes usually have to be tossed after 400 to 500 miles.) Replace your shoes when the tread begins to wear thin or when the sides start to cave inward or outward. Walking shoes may sound like a marketing conspiracy hatched by shoeindustry executives. After all, it's only walking — won't any pair of sneakers suffice? Actually, the concept of a walking shoe is a valid one. Walking shoes need to be more flexible than running shoes because you bend your feet more when you walk, and you push off from your toes with more oomph. Also, because your heels bear most of your weight when you walk, you need a firm, stable heel counter, the part of the shoe that wraps around your heel to keep your foot in place. If you plan to hike or walk over rugged terrain, look for a walking shoe with treaded soles and added heel and ankle support. If you're focusing on speed walking or high mileage, go for a little more cushioning in the midsole, the area between the tread and the inside of the shoe. Walking the right way Okay, we lied to you: There actually is more to walking than simply putting one foot in front of the other. The biggest mistake walkers make is bending forward, a sure way to develop problems in your lower back, neck, and hips. Your posture should be naturally tall. You needn't force yourself to be ramrod straight, but neither should you slouch, overarch your back, or lean too far forward from your hips. Relax your shoulders, widen your chest, and pull your abdominals gently inward. Keep your head and chin up and focus straight ahead. Meanwhile, keep your hands relaxed and cupped gently, and swing your arms so that they brush past your body. On the upswing, your hand should be level with your breast bone; on the downswing, your hand should brush against your hip. Keep your hips loose and relaxed. Your feet should land firmly, heel first. Roll through your heel to your arch, then to the ball of your foot, and then to your toes. Push off from your toes and the ball of your foot.Although walking is the most basic of all fitness activities, novice fitness walkers can still benefit from the following pointers: Increase your workout time gradually. Most people can start off with five 10- to 20-minute walking sessions a week; after about a month, they can increase each workout by 2 or 3 minutes per week until walking 30 to 45 minutes is comfortable. (Five days a week may sound like a lot, but an almost-daily walk makes it easier to get in the habit.) Walk as fast as you comfortably can. If you walk very fast — at a 12-minute-mile to 15-minute-mile pace — you can burn twice as many calories as when you walk at a 20-minute-mile pace. You may not be able to move at such supersonic speeds in the beginning, but as you get fit, you can mix in some fast-paced intervals. (For details about interval training.) If you're walking on the shoulder of a road, walk against traffic so you can watch cars approach. On sidewalks or trails, walk any old way you want. Add some hills. Walking over hilly terrain shapes your butt and thighs and burns extra calories (about 30 percent more calories than walking on flat terrain, depending, of course, on the grade of the hills). Sneak in a walk whenever you can. Leave your car at home and hoof it to the train station. Take a 15-minute walk during your lunch break. Traverse the airport on foot rather than on that automatic walking belt. It all adds up.

Like walking, running is a workout that you can take with you anywhere. You don't need a rack on your car or a suitcase full of equipment; you just open the door and go. Plus, as any pathological runner will tell you, nothing is quite as satisfying as getting a good run under your belt. You work up a great sweat, you burn lots of calories, and your muscles feel pleasantly invigorated after you finish. No single type of exercise is better than all the rest. It's merely a question of what's best for you. Many runners develop frequent, chronic injuries. Many people have joints that simply will not tolerate all that pounding. If you're not built to run, don't argue with your body. You can get in great condition in other ways. And if you're a beginner, hold off on running until you've built up stamina and strength. Essential running gear Although you can spend hundreds of dollars on spiffy warm-ups, tights, and tops, the only equipment that's truly essential for running is a good pair of shoes (although women will want a supportive jogging bra, too). Be prepared to spend at least $50 to $60 a pair, but know that a hefty price tag doesn't always correspond to the best shoe. The shoe that's best for you depends on your weight, the shape of your foot, your running style, and any special problems you may have, such as weak ankles or bad knees. Try on several models at the store, and take each one for a test drive around the mall or at least run a couple laps around the store. Your running shoes should be fairly flexible, especially across the ball of the foot. Hold the shoe at both ends and bend it; it should break right at the ball of the foot. You want cushioning, but not so much that you can't feel your foot hitting the ground. Look for a stable heel counter (the part of the shoe that wraps around your heel to keep your foot in place). If your foot slides around a lot, that can mean trouble down the road. Running the right way Runners have a habit of looking directly at the ground, almost as if they can't bear to see what's coming next. Keeping your head down throws your upperbody posture off-kilter and can lead to upper-back and neck pain. Lift your head and focus your eyes straight ahead. Relax your shoulders, keep your chest lifted, and pull your abdominal muscles in tightly. Don't overarch your back and stick your butt out; that's one of the main reasons runners get back and hip pain. Keep your arms close to your body, and swing them forward and back rather than across your body. Don't clench your fists. Pretend you're holding a butterfly in each hand; you don't want your butterflies to escape, but you don't want to crush them, either. Lift your front knee and extend your back leg. Don't shuffle along like you're wearing cement boots. Land heel first and roll through the entire length of your foot. Push off from the balls of your feet instead of running flat-footed 150 Part III: Getting to the Heart of the Matter and pounding off your heels. Otherwise, your feet and legs are going to cry uncle long before your cardiovascular system does. If you experience pain in your ankles, knees, or lower back, stop running for a while. If you don't, you could end up having to sit on the sidelines for months. Running tips for rookies These tips help you get fit and avoid injury. Start by alternating periods of walking with periods of running. For example, try two minutes of walking and one minute of running. Gradually decrease your walking intervals until you can run continuously for 20 minutes. If you have the inclination, you can build from there. Of course, sticking with a walk-run routine is fine; you're less likely to injure yourself that way. Vary your pace. Different paces work your heart, lungs, and legs in different ways. Experiment with the techniques described in Chapter 8. Always run against traffic when running on the shoulder of a road. This allows you to see oncoming cars and dive for the side of the road, if necessary. If you're running on steeply banked (angled away from the center line) country roads and the road is flat, you can run in the middle of the road to save wear and tear on your legs. But as you head up or down hills, get as far over on the shoulder (that is, away from the road) as possible to avoid speeding cars mowing you down. Consider carrying a lightweight cell phone for emergencies. Don't increase your mileage by more than 10 percent a week. If you run 5 miles a week and want to increase, aim to do 51/2 miles the following week. Jumping from 5 miles to 6 miles doesn't sound like a big deal, but studies show that if you increase your mileage more than 10 percent, you set yourself up for injury. Bicycling: Road and Mountain Talk to a group of cyclists and, chances are, you're talking to a group of exrunners. Cycling is perfect for people who can't take the relentless pounding of running or find the slow pace a real drag. Cycling is the best way to cover a lot of ground quickly. Even a novice can easily build up to a 20-mile ride. Cycling can be a hassle. You can't just grab your shoes and head out the door. You need your helmet, water bottle, gloves, sunscreen, and glasses. And even with all your protective gear, you can never be too cautious. Cycling is a lowimpact sport — unless you happen to impact the ground, a car, a tree, a rut, or another cyclist.

To protect your knees from injury, position your seat correctly (ask your salesperson for advice) and pedal at an easy cadence. Cadence refers to the number of revolutions per minute that you pedal. Inexperienced cyclists tend to use a higher gear than they can handle, which forces them to turn the pedals in slow motion; their legs tire prematurely, their knees ache, and they cheat themselves out of a good workout. Set your bike's gear so you're pedaling at a comfortable cadence. Road cycling can wreak havoc on your lower back because you're in a crouched position for so long. Relax your upper body and keep your arms loose. Grasp your handlebars with the same tension that you'd hold a child's hand when you cross the street. Pedal in smooth circles rather than simply mashing the pedals downward. Imagine that you have a bed of nails in your shoes, and you have to pedal without stomping on the nails. Cycling tips for rookies You can learn a lot about cycling — and get faster in a jif — by riding with a club or friends who have more experience. Here are some pointers to start your cycling career: Remember that you are a vehicle and are required to follow the rules of the road. Ride with traffic, not against it. Stop at all signs and lights, and use those hand signals you learned in driver's ed. Don't trust a single car, ever. Assume that the driver doesn't see you, even if he happens to be staring you in the face. When you go off-road, start on wide fire roads rather than narrow "single-track" trails that require technical skills. And don't think that you're immune to injury because there are no cars. More crashes happen on mountain trails than on the road because there are more obstacles and riders get careless and cocky. Head into a turn at a slow enough pace that you maintain control, and never let your eyes wander from the road or trail. Never squeeze the brakes — particularly the front brake — with a lot of pressure. You'll go flying over the handlebars, a maneuver known as an endo, and go right into a face plant, a maneuver that we think is self-explanatory.Exercising Outdoors 153 In-Line Skating In 1980, Rollerblade introduced a new kind of skate: Instead of two wheels at the toe and two wheels at the heel, the four wheels were positioned in a single-file line. This was the biggest innovation in skating since a 16th-century Dutchman patterned the first pair of roller skates after ice skates. Now in-line skating — often called Rollerblading — is the skate of choice for more than 15 million people. Skating is fun because it isn't as linear as running, walking, and cycling. You can curve, turn, glide, sprint, and spin. Skating is also a terrific tush toner because you push your legs out to the side, which works several seldom-used hip muscles. Skating is a good calorie burner, too. But in-line skating is also dangerous. About 270,000 skaters per year wind up at the doctor or emergency room with injuries. Liz got a first-hand look at one of these injuries not long ago. While running over the 59th Street Bridge in New York City, Liz spotted a woman walking in bare feet and sobbing. The woman's entire left side was so bloody that she appeared to have been mauled by a tiger. It turns out the woman had attempted to skate over sharp metal teeth on the road — teeth designed to provide traction for cars during icy conditions in winter. Most skaters use more common sense than that, but injuries are still common because the sport requires so much balance and concentration. Plus, stopping on in-line skates is darn tough. (See "Skating the right way," later in this chapter, for stopping tips.)

There are 650 muscles in your body. We are happy to report that you don't need to memorize all of them. Consider, for example, the inferior retinaculum of the long extensor of your big toe. We don't want you to remember that one. In fact, we don't even know that one — we had to look it up in our anatomy book. If you have any desire to find out more about that muscle, shut this book and apply to medical school. Meanwhile, in this chapter, we tell you about the 20 or so muscles that any conscientious exerciser should know. What's the point? For one thing, you won't need an interpreter when a trainer, video instructor, or fellow gym member says, "Let's do lats and pecs today." Before you know it, you may be saying stuff like that, too. And you'll sound really impressive — like wine aficionados who say, "This chardonnay has a superior bouquet." But more importantly, if you can name your major muscles and understand how each one operates, you can get better results from your workout program. You'll understand, for example, how certain exercises can help you prevent lower-back pain. You'll understand why you should do several different shoulder exercises, rather than just one. And you'll be sure to perform your exercises properly. For example, if you know where your biceps are, you'll realize exactly where you should feel the tension — and you can adjust your form if you don't feel tension in the right spot. With many weight-training exercises, it's easy to emphasize the wrong muscle if you don't understand the purpose of the move. If you simply hop on a machine and pull some lever without knowing which muscle to focus on, you may be cheating yourself out of a good workout. Finally, knowing about all your major muscle groups helps you get a more complete and balanced workout. You'll know not to leave any muscle group out.

Shoulders Strong shoulders are the key to building a strong upper body. Just about every exercise you can do for your chest and back involves your shoulders, too. If your shoulders are weak, you really limit the amount of weight you can use in the rest of your upper-body repertoire. Deltoids Given name: Deltoids Street name: Delts Whereabouts: Your delts wrap completely around the tops of your arms . Cup your hand over your shoulder and you get the idea. Now swing your arm around in a circle, raise it up above your head, and then swing it forward and backward. You can see what a versatile muscle your shoulder is. The front portion of the shoulder muscle is referred to as the anterior delt, the side is called the medial delt, and the back is called the rear or posterior delt. Go ahead, toss those terms around and amaze your friends.

Job description: Your delts help your arms move in a wide range of directions. The training payoff: You'll never have to wear shoulder pads if, heaven forbid, they ever come back in style. Also, strengthening your shoulders can help you avoid injuries such as shoulder dislocations or muscle tears. And with strong shoulders, you have no trouble putting that useless "waist trimmer" gadget that you bought for $19.95 on the top shelf in the closet. Special tips: We tend to like free weights better than machines for strengthening the shoulders. Although most shoulder-press machines have improved in recent years, many other shoulder contraptions, especially lateralraise machines, tend to be difficult to adjust and uncomfortable to use. Also, machines aren't made for every shoulder movement. For example, no specific machine mimics the front shoulder raise. It's important to target the front, middle, and back of your shoulders, as well as the delts as a whole, so make it a point to master several dumbbell exercises. Our favorite exercises: Dumbbell shoulder press, dumbbell lateral raise, dumbbell front raise, and dumbbell back delt fly Rotator cuff Given name: Rotator cuff Street name: Rotators Whereabouts: Four small muscles beneath your shoulder together, they're called your rotator cuff. Job description: Your rotator-cuff muscles hold your arm in its socket. You use these muscles to rotate the shoulder joint, such as when throwing and catching. Baseball pitchers are constantly sidelined with rotator-cuff injuries. The training payoff: If you have weak rotators, you can damage them simply by carrying a briefcase or reaching across the table for Rice Krispies Treats — throwing a 90 mph fastball is not a prerequisite for injury . By making a special effort to strengthen these commonly injured muscles, you're far less likely to tear or strain them. Special tips: In addition to doing rotator-cuff exercises, work your shoulders in a variety of directions. Your rotators are put into action whenever your deltoids are working; if your delts are weak and you do a heavy upper-body lift, you may do some serious rotator damage. If you have chronic shoulder pain, check with your orthopedist to see if you've injured your rotator cuff. Sometimes rotator tears can be corrected with exercise; other times, they require surgery.

Our favorite exercises: Internal and external rotation, performed with an exercise band, a dumbbell, or a weight plate, or on a cable crossover machine Back Neglecting your back muscles is tempting because you don't face them in the mirror every day. But these muscles are just as important as the muscles in the front of your body, particularly when it comes to injury prevention. We know a man who injured his back while putting on his underwear in the health-club locker room. He was lying on the floor stark naked for a few hours before he let the staff members call a nurse. Trainers had repeatedly reminded him to strengthen his lower-back muscles and abdominals. After that incident, he finally listened. Trapezius Given name: Trapezius Street name: Traps Whereabouts: Your trapezius is a fairly large, kite-shaped muscle that spans up into your neck, across your shoulders, and down to the center of your back.

Job description: Your trapezius enables you to shrug your shoulders. This muscle is also involved when you lift your arm, such as when hailing a cab. The training payoff: A toned trapezius adds shape to your shoulders and upper back. Strengthening this muscle may also alleviate the neck and shoulder pain you may get if you sit at a desk all day or if your phone is a permanent appendage to your ear. Special tips: Give your trapezius extra attention if you often carry a knapsack or heavy bag over your shoulder. Our favorite exercises: Shrug or shoulder roll with a barbell, two dumbbells, or — if your neck is extremely weak and tight — no weight at all Latissimus dorsi Given name: Latissimus dorsi Street name: Lats (Note: Don't make the mistake of saying "laterals," as some less-informed, bookwormish exercisers do.) Whereabouts: Feel the widest part of your back just behind your armpit — you've just found your latissimus dorsi, your largest back muscle. This muscle runs the entire length of your back, from below your shoulders down to your lower back.

Job description: Your lats enable you to pull, like when you open a door against the wind or drag your Great Dane into the vet's office. The training payoff: Well-toned lats make your hips and waist appear smaller by adding shape and width to your upper body. If you play sports — especially a racquet sport, golf, or hockey — strengthening your lats will enable you to power the ball or puck quite a bit further. Runners, walkers, and cyclists also should focus on their lats to help counteract that tendency toward rounded shoulders, which are the result of weak rhomboids (see the following section) and other muscles of the upper and middle back, as well as the result of tight delts (discussed in the "Deltoids" section) and pecs (see the "Chest (the Pectorals)" section). Special tips: When you do lat exercises, think of your arms simply as a link between your back and the bar or dumbbell. Focus on working your lats, not your arms. Our favorite exercises: Lat pull-down machine, dumbbell row, dumbbell pullover, T-bar row, seated cable row, chin-up, and pull-up Rhomboids Given name: Rhomboids Street name: None. Almost no one talks about them. (However, we did once hear them referred to as the "rheumatoids," a term we thought was better suited for an octogenarian garage band.) Whereabouts: Your rhomboids are a small, rectangular group of muscles at the center of your back, hidden beneath your lower trapezius (refer to Figure 12-4). Job description: Your rhomboids pull your shoulder blades together so you maintain good posture. The training payoff: With strong rhomboids, you're less likely to hunch your shoulders forward. Special tips: Focus on your rhomboids to avoid poor posture and potential injury. Our favorite exercises: Chin-up and dumbbell back delt fly Erector spinae Given name: Erector spinae Street name: Lower back Whereabouts: Your erector spinae run the entire length of your spine, but it's the lower third of this muscle group that you strengthen when you perform the exercises we mention later in this section. The rest of this muscle group gets worked when you do upper-back exercises. Figure 12-5 shows where your erector spinae are located. Job description: Your lower-back muscles are responsible for straightening your spine — for example, when you stand up after tying your shoes. They also work in tandem with your abdominals to keep your spine stable when you move the rest of your body, like when you're sitting in your car and you reach around for something in the back seat. The training payoff: About 80 percent of adult Americans experience back pain at some point in their lives. You can prevent much of this pain by devoting equal time to strengthening your lower back and abdominal muscles. Strong lower-back muscles are also very important for posture.

Chest (the Pectorals) The fibers of your chest muscles spread out like a fan, connecting to your arms, ribs, collar bone (clavical), and breast bone (sternum). For this reason, your chest muscles respond well when you work them from a variety of angles. For example, you can do chest exercises while lying flat on your back on a bench, reclining at various angles, sitting upright, standing, or lying facedown (like when you do push-ups). Ask a trainer to show you several chest exercises so you can vary your workouts. Given name: Pectorals Street name: Pecs Whereabouts: Place your hand on your chest as if you're pledging allegiance to the flag. You've found your pecs.

Job description: Thanks to your pecs you can push — a shopping cart, a lawn mover, or some jerk standing in your way. You also use your pecs to wrap your arms around something, like when you give your mom a bear hug.

The training payoff: With strong pecs, you look great in tight t-shirts. You also need strong chest muscles for sports like tennis, golf, and football. Special tips: For women — it's important to understand that your pecs are not your breasts; in fact they reside directly underneath your breast tissue. However, toning your pecs can lift your breasts and make them appear firmer. For men — don't become obsessed with bench pressing to the point of excluding all other exercises. Men with overdeveloped chest muscles and wimpy legs resemble hard-boiled eggs on toothpicks. Besides, doing too much chest work sets you up for shoulder injuries. Our favorite exercises: Bench press, dumbbell fly, push-up, and incline dumbbell press.

Arms Take a survey of today's TV stars, fashion models, and music artists, and you can see that firm arm muscles are in style. Even department-store mannequins now have toned arms. Be sure to give your front and rear arm muscles equal time; if one of these muscle groups is disproportionately stronger than the other, you're at greater risk for elbow injuries.

Biceps Given name: Biceps Street name: Bi(s) or guns Whereabouts: Your biceps are the two muscles at the front of your upper arm — the ones that pop up when you flex like a bodybuilder. Job description: Your biceps are responsible for bending your elbow. When you pick up this book or when you turn the pages, you use your biceps. The training payoff: With strong biceps, lifting a stack of newspapers or carrying an armload of wood is easier. Your biceps also help out your back muscles when you pull a really stubborn weed out of your garden. Plus, strong biceps make you look buff.

Special tips: Many people have sloppy posture when they do biceps exercises — they rock their bodies back and forth to hoist the weight up. Not only is this posture dangerous for your lower back, but it also makes life too easy for your biceps. Pay special attention to form on bicep exercises, and don't use more weight than you can handle. Our favorite exercises: Dumbbell biceps curl, concentration curl, barbell biceps curl, and machine arm curl Triceps Given name: Triceps Street name: Tri(s) Whereabouts: Your triceps are located at the back of your upper arm (refer to Figure 12-7). Job description: Your triceps do the opposite of what your biceps do; that is, your triceps straighten your elbow. Your triceps help out your chest muscles when you push something, like your 1966 Volkswagen Bug that has stalled at an intersection. The training payoff: Triceps exercises help firm up bingo arms. That's when the backs of your arms flap loosely away from the bones — a condition common among people whose main form of physical activity is playing bingo. Special tips: The triceps make up two-thirds of your upper-arm size, so if you want a nice pair of arms, work these muscles. Working your triceps is especially important if you often hold a briefcase or handbag while your arm is straight. If your triceps are weak — and that's common because these muscles don't get much work in daily life — you may be prone to elbow pain. Our favorite exercises: Triceps kickback, bench dip, triceps press-down, and triceps-extension machine or dumbbells/barbells. Forearm muscles Given name: Wrist extensors and flexors Street name: Wrist or forearm muscles Whereabouts: These muscles run from the bottom of your elbow to your wrist.

Job description: Your forearm muscles bend and move your wrists. They're also a link between your upper body and any barbell, lever, or dumbbell you move. If you don't have the wrist strength to grip a barbell, you're certainly not going to be able to bench-press, even if your chest muscles are strong. The training payoff: Powerful wrist muscles give you a stronger grip for weight lifting. Wrist strength also can help prevent or alleviate tennis elbow and carpal tunnel syndrome — a painful irritation of wrist nerves resulting from repetitive motions such as typing or certain assemblyline tasks, such as tightening a bolt with a wrench. Special tips: To ensure that you develop adequate wrist strength, wrap your hand firmly around the barbells or dumbbells you use. Our favorite exercises: Dumbbell wrist curl and reverse wrist curl.

If your rear end and hips are larger than you'd like them to be, don't be afraid to strengthen these muscles with weights. With the right workout program, these muscles can look firmer and more shapely, not bigger and bulkier. Also, strengthening your butt and hip muscles can help prevent hip and lower-back injuries. If your job requires you to sit on your rear end all day, doing exercises that target these muscles is a good idea. Gluteus maximus Given name: Gluteus maximus Street name: Glutes, buns, or butt Whereabouts: The largest muscle in your body — as if you need anyone to tell you that. Your two glutes (left and right cheeks) span the entire width of your derriere.

Job description: Your glutes extend your hips and help you jump, climb stairs and hills, and straighten your leg behind you. You also use your gluteus maximus when you stand up from a sitting position. The training payoff: Training your glutes can lift your butt, make it rounder, and give it more shape. You also need your glutes to get off the couch so you can go work out. Special tips: Some glute exercises, such as the squat and the lunge (elongated variations of deep knee bends), can be hard on your knees, so pay extra attention to your form. When you bend your knees, your kneecaps should move in the direction that your toes are facing, and they should not shoot out past your toes. Our favorite exercises: Squat, lunge, and leg-press machine.

Hip abductors Given name: Hip abductors Street name: Outer thighs or outer hip Whereabouts: The meatiest part of the side of your hips. Job description: Your abductors help you slide your leg out to the side, like when you go skating or step aside so someone can get past you. These muscles also help your gluteus maximus (or butt) rotate your hips outward.

Legs Keep in mind that, if all goes well, your legs will be carrying you from here to there for the rest of your life. So treat them with respect. By strengthening your leg muscles, you can head off many common knee and ankle injuries. And by staying healthy, of course, you can stay active. You can work out more and develop lean, toned legs that power you up a hill and look good in shorts. Quadriceps Given name: Quadriceps Street name: Quads Whereabouts: Your quadriceps are the four muscles at the front of each thigh . Job description: Your quadriceps straighten your knee. The training payoff: You need strong quads for walking, running, climbing, skiing, skating, hopping, skipping, and jumping. Keeping your quads strong can help prevent knee problems. (If you already have knee pain, check with your doctor to find out which exercises are best for you.) Special tips: Don't worry if you feel an intense burning sensation when you do the leg . This is one of the few exercises that completely isolates the quads, which causes them to tire quickly. Waste products like lactic acid flood into the muscles, causing you to really feel the burn. Our favorite exercises: Squat, lunge, leg press, and leg-extension machine Hamstrings Given name: Hamstrings Street name: Hams Whereabouts: Your hamstrings are the three muscles at the back of your thigh . Job description: Your hamstrings work in opposition to your quadriceps; in other words, your hamstrings bend the knee. They also help out your glutes when you move from a sitting to a standing position.

Gastrocnemius and soleus Given names: Gastrocnemius and soleus Street name: Calves Whereabouts: Your gastrocnemius, also called your gastroc, is the large diamond-shaped muscle that gives shape to the back of your lower legs. (To see precisely what the gastroc looks like, pedal behind any top-notch cyclist.) The soleus resides underneath the gastroc (see Figure 12-10). Job description: Your calf muscles allow you to stand on your tiptoes and spring off the ground whenever you jump for joy. Gastrocnemius Soleus Tibialis Anterior Figure 12-10: Your lowerleg muscles. Your Muscles: Love 'Em or Lose 'Em The training payoff: Strong and shapely calves don't just look good; they also give you staying power when you take those long, romantic walks or wait in a three-hour line for Garth Brooks tickets. Plus, you need strong calves for dancing, jumping, running, and hopping. Special tips: With calf exercises, some people find it more effective to use slightly lighter weights and do a few more repetitions — say, up to 25 — than with most other muscle groups. The muscle tissue in your calves is made specifically for endurance (walking and standing), so it takes more repetitions to reach the deepest fibers. Our favorite exercises: Standing calf raise, seated calf raise, and standingcalf-raise machine Tibialis anterior Given name: Tibialis anterior Street name: Shins Whereabouts: The tibialis anterior is the largest of several muscles that run from the top of your foot up the lower leg to the outside of the shin bone, near the knee .

Job description: Your shin muscles enable you to pull your toes toward your shin, as when you pick up your foot when walking or running. The training payoff: Shin splints — throbbing pain at the front of your ankles caused by any sort of irritation or inflammation in the shins — are fairly common among walkers, runners, dancers, and aerobicizers who overdo it .

Ways To Stay Fit And Healthy

Staying fit and healthy plays an important role in our life. People neglect their health because of the hectic daily schedules but there are little things that you can do each day that will add to being healthy and fit.One should get annual physical check up to make sure everything is as it should be. There is no harm getting regular check ups as it's good for your own body. Do breast or testicular self-exams and get suspicious moles checked out. Getting exams regularly benefits you because if and when something is abnormal, you will get to know about it timely and can consult with your doctor.

Getting enough sleep is necessary to stay fit and healthy, many of us do not get enough.

Lack of sleep affects our physical and mental health tremendously. It also affects metabolism, mood, concentration, memory, motor skills, stress hormones and even the immune system and cardiovascular health.

Sleep allows the body to heal, repair and rejuvenate.

Exercise is important for being fit and healthy. One should walk for few minutes everyday to stay fit.

It also improves circulation and body awareness and can help combat depression.

Cardiovascular exercise helps to strengthen the heart and lungs, strength training helps to strengthen the muscles and stretching helps to reduce the risk of injury by increasing flexibility.

Eat lots of fresh fruits, vegetables,and whole grains to stay healthy and fit. Also include lean sources of protein such as poultry, fish, tofu and beans into your diet.

One should eat a balanced meal and not overeat. Junk foods like burgers, pizza and those that are highly processed and contain artificial sweeteners should be strictly avoided.

One should have healthy breakfast as it keeps you energetic and fuelled for optimal mental and physical performance. Eating breakfast helps to maintain stable blood sugar levels and a healthy weight because you are less likely to overindulge later in the day.

Drink plenty of water as it helps in keeping our bodies hydrated and to maintain a healthy body. It is the natural cleanser for our organs and digestive system. Water also helps in flushing toxins out through the skin and urine.

Stress is not good as it harms the body and can cause a myriad of problems, from heart trouble to digestive problems. Exercise, meditation, doing what you love, appropriate boundaries, spirituality, being in nature and enjoyable hobbies helps to alleviate the harmful effects of stress on the body.

Don't overwork and take breaks and surround yourself with people who support you.